Fat Tactics

Fat Tactics

The Rhetoric and Structure of the Fat Acceptance Movement

By Erec Smith

LEXINGTON BOOKS
Lanham • Boulder • New York • London

Published by Lexington Books
An imprint of The Rowman & Littlefield Publishing Group, Inc.
4501 Forbes Boulevard, Suite 200, Lanham, Maryland 20706
www.rowman.com

6 Tinworth Street, London SE11 5AL

British Library Cataloguing in Publication Information Available

Library of Congress Cataloging-in-Publication Data

Names: Smith, Erec, author.
Title: Fat tactics : the rhetoric and structure of the fat acceptance movement / Erec Smith.
Description: Lanham : Lexington Books, [2019] | Includes bibliographical references and index.
Identifiers: LCCN 2018048500 (print) | LCCN 2018049192 (ebook) | ISBN 9781498531177 (electronic) | ISBN 9781498531160 (cloth : alk. paper)
Subjects: LCSH: Discrimination against overweight persons. | Obesity--Social aspects.
Classification: LCC RC628 (ebook) | LCC RC628 .S6413 2019 (print) | DDC 362.1963/98--dc23
LC record available at https://lccn.loc.gov/2018048500

∞™ The paper used in this publication meets the minimum requirements of American National Standard for Information Sciences Permanence of Paper for Printed Library Materials, ANSI/NISO Z39.48-1992.

Printed in the United States of America

Contents

Preface

The other day, a new Facebook acquaintance asked me why I was involved in the Fat Acceptance movement—particularly, a Fat Acceptance Facebook page—and why I considered it "awesome." My answer:

a. I know and have seen that health is something one can have at a variety of sizes. Unfortunately, convincing others can be difficult. So, I was delighted to see that many people have dedicated their time, intellect, and overall brilliance to this endeavor.
b. I believe that beauty comes in all sizes, and am happy to see a community that not only believes this but PROVES it.
c. I think through my standpoint and intellectual interests, I can contribute to the mission of Fat Acceptance.

I then discussed my own intersectionality and how it may inform my participation in the movement.

Although I meant what I wrote, I felt odd about it. As "not-fat"[1] and male, I had a keen feeling that any reasons I gave for my interests in Fat Acceptance may be met with rolled eyes and seen as less authentic than those of fat people, specifically fat women. What's more, my race raised other questions about my perceived interest in the movement. On one hand, I suddenly felt like some kind of colonizer; an archeologist living among the natives as authentically as possible but knowing he'll be able to go back to his cozy upscale home at the end of it all. On the other hand, I felt the potential for misrecognition based on contemporary myths that black men covet fat women. Although I already knew that my interest in Fat Studies and Fat Acceptance would and should be analyzed, I never welcomed the difficulty and pain that could potentially accompany this analysis.

What is the motivation, after all? From where does passion for something derive? I can say that I recognize and empathize with the pain of stigmatization. I've weathered privileged people's attempts to humiliate or silence me based on my differences. But there are many groups that deal with this, not just fat people. So, why have I gravitated toward the Fat Acceptance Movement instead of some other marginalized demographic . . . like my own?

The honest truth is difficult and multifaceted. This multiplicity is reflected in the concept of diversity. My stints as a diversity officer and diversity committee chair led me to Fat Studies and Fat Acceptance, and I explored it with both intrigue and admiration. I noticed an inherent critique of hegemony and the determination to speak truth to power in this movement. I discerned the challenges the movement presents to unknowing, sheltered, and, unfortunately, powerful people who define beauty or health based on traditional and often Eurocentric preferences and questionable information. I recognized the intersectionality of this movement: fat stigma affects people from all walks of life in differing ways that are inherently informative and interesting. Lastly, I recognize the beauty, bravery, and brilliance of its scholars and activists. The Greeks had a term, *kalos kai agathos*, which is "an ideal that unites physical beauty and moral value in a human being"[2] I recognize this concept throughout the movement, and I am drawn to it as both a scholar and ally. The confluence of all these things have piqued my interest in this movement as a rhetorician; the rhetorical criticism, countercultural standpoint, and challenge to grand narratives of beauty and virtue are central to Fat Acceptance.

However, I must be careful to avoid becoming a new manifestation of the kind of privilege Peggy McIntosh called "foolish, ridiculous, infantile or dangerous by contrast."[3]

Thus, I start with a self-assessment of my subject position in the context of Fat Studies and Fat Activism. Marilyn Wann, in her foreword to *The Fat Studies Reader*, suggests that all scholars and activists of the Fat Acceptance movement realize our subject positions in relation to the Fat Acceptance movement. That is, who are we and how do our past and present experiences affect what we say about this movement? I took this advice seriously and realized that my stance within this community is more complicated than I initially thought. Although my subject position is necessarily intersectional (as is everyone's), I realized that the best way to understand it, for myself and others, may be to break it up into its constituent parts, discuss each part individually, and explore how their confluence informs my views.

Perhaps most significantly, I am not fat by societal standards. Many liberation movements have encountered the beneficent outsider: that privileged person willing to fight for the causes of the underprivileged. Often, this person does more harm than good, an occurrence frequent enough to induce suspicion in his or her underprivileged cohort. The privileged activist may even have a savior complex of sorts. As a non-fat person who considers himself a fat activist and Fat Studies scholar, I must be cognizant of these trends.

I know that I must avoid speaking *for* fat people instead of supporting them when they speak for themselves. I can support causes of fat liberation, write about my position in the Fat Acceptance movement, and give my insights in an attempt to inform people of the various perspectives within this field, but I am not some lofty, empowered figure that this movement *needs* in any significant way. Although I see myself as an activist, I am here to take a backseat in assisting this movement and will only take a front seat if called to. Ultimately, I must emphasize a need to *listen* and act accordingly to those who *most* embody this movement.

Secondly, I identify as a cisgender male, giving me double-privilege (at least) within the Fat Acceptance movement. This movement consists mostly of women and always has. Fat men do suffer from weight discrimination but not nearly as much as women. A fat man can be a leading man, an athlete (look at any lineman in the NFL), even president of the United States. Fat women have come along a bit regarding pop cultural acceptance, but do not share the societal luxury of their male counterparts.

Race also plays a role. As a Black person in America, I have suffered from various manifestations of racial discrimination. Despite a more improved racial climate, race relations are still problematic. Thus, I can relate significantly to the irritation and frustration induced by those in society who do not realize their privilege. Perhaps this is exacerbated by my upbringing in a predominately White environment, which made me an even more distinct and obvious minority and, therefore, empathetic to others who may have felt the same.

For many White Americans, being thin is proof that one does, indeed, deserve to be White. Perhaps—and more in line with the thoughts of fat scholars like Amy Farrell, Paul Campos, Peter Stearns, and others—thinness has been usurped by White culture as a way to separate itself from cultures who do not stigmatize fat or, completely adversely, praise fat bodies. Either way, it seems that as a Black man, I am "allowed" to be fat and admire fat bodies, which leads to a very important corollary: a fat White person or even a white ally of the Fat Acceptance movement is typically NOT acceptable and would be considered a disgrace to his race—a race of which the hegemonic power in this society largely consists.

My original scholarly interests lie in the field of rhetoric. I am interested in the tropes used within interpretive communities to either support or deride certain modes of thought or action. Thus, my interests in the Fat Acceptance Movement are not just about activism. I want to explore the symbols of Fat Acceptance, Fat Admiration, and anti-Fat Activism. I also want to explore the stories within the Fat Acceptance community that help explain the movement to those unaware of its existence, those apprehensive to join, and those against the movement for whatever reasons (cultural, financial, etc.). More directly, I am interested in preferred Discourses within the Fat Acceptance community. Ultimately, I am interested in the salient aspects and efficacies of Fat Acceptance activists.

Do my race, upbringing, weight, sex, and occupation create a specific lens through which I see this movement or a particular filter through which I hear it? Of course it does. What my own personal intersectionality suggests, however, is that there is no one way to see things even for a single person. The eclecticism of the movement, itself—regarding race, sex, gender, socioeconomic status, age, and so forth—suggests that any single take on the movement is just that: a single take. I can only speak as a not-fat, African-American, male rhetorician. However, that doesn't mean my viewpoint within Fat Acceptance cannot be informative to others. What's more, I think the opinions of readers will be very informative to me. I look forward to finding out.

NOTES

1. I would not say I am thin, but I am not fat by societal standards. Thus, I frequently use the adjective "non-fat" as a self-descriptor.
2. M. A. Dürrigl, "Kalokagathia—beauty is more than just external appearance," *Journal of Cosmetic Dermatology* 1.1 (2002), Web. 19 Jun. 2012, 208, http://jrscience.wcp.muohio.edu/humans_web_04/beauty/beauty.pdf.
3. Peggy McIntosh, "White Privilege and Male Privilege: A Personal Account of Coming to See Correspondences through Work in Women's Studies," *Privilege: A Reader*, ed. Michael S. Kimmel and Abby L. Ferber. 1st ed. (New York: Basic Books, 2003), 155. Print.

Introduction

The "Spirit" of Fat Acceptance

A zeitgeist clearly exists within the Fat Acceptance Movement. This spirit moves through several circles, including those of activism, fashion, and academia. However, all these circles share an almost spiritual motivation to work for and perpetuate fat pride.

In "The Co-Construction of Self and Organization: Evoking Organizational Spirituality," Diane F. Witmer suggests that an organic spirituality often develops within organizations that work to protect, support, and empower its members.[1] She writes,

> In order for the concept of organizational spirituality to inform scholarly research, it is important to tease the concepts of *religiosity,* spiritual *belief* and matters of *faith* from the snarled literature. The question is not whether human agents believe in a God, or gods, or oneness with nature, or hobgoblins, nor whether the religious path is Christian, Buddhist, Druid, or Wiccan, but that there is some power that is greater than mere humanity, and that a noncorporeal essence imbues humanness. Human understanding or acknowledgement of that power does not create it, nor does human denial destroy it. It simply *is.*[2]

It seems that activism, aesthetic pride in the fat body, the sharing of narratives of oppression and triumph, the laughter and the tears (sometime simultaneously) may induce an affect that smacks of something "greater than mere humanity." I see it in the stories told and the interconnectedness these stories expose. Narrative is often the glue that connects individuals into larger groups and organizations. Narratives serve as explanations of interconnectedness and intersectionality. They are beacons that let people know they are not alone; others share their stories and emotions. Narratives show us that a seemingly impossible triumph over societal biases and oppressions is possible and that one need not do it alone. Fat activist Golda Schein, during a "Body Love Wellness" teleconference series, began every call by asking its featured speakers to give their "origin stories"—the narratives of how they discovered and entered into Fat Acceptance. Schein was wise to do this and wise to use such a term. ("Origin Story" is the common way to describe stories of how superheroes acquired their powers.) She may have realized that these stories did not just provide ethos for the speakers; they provided a deep connection among the speakers and members. The spirit of the Fat Acceptance Movement is in its stories.

The ultimate creation of this spirit, however, may come from cocreating these stories. Interconnectedness is already apparent through individual stories, but as we come together at conferences, social events, internet forums, and Facebook groups, we begin to "write" these stories together. If individual stories are powerful, stories created by multiple "authors" would create a zeitgeist previously unimagined.

Of course, issues of communication should be considered. Regardless of intersectionality, the cultural, sexual, or socioeconomic experiences of one person may be foreign to those of another. I believe it is this spirit and faith in interconnectedness and recognition of the interdependence of the members that can assuage any disquietude that may result. The key may be found in finding the common feelings members may have. This is easier said than done.

In *Nonviolent Communication: A Language of Life*, Marshall B. Rosenberg expresses that the key to compassionate and effective speech, "Nonviolent Communication" (NVC), in the face of conflict is through four components: observation, feeling, needs, and request. He writes,

> First, we observe what is actually happening in a situation: what are we observing others saying or doing that is either enriching or not enriching our life? The trick is to be able to articulate this observation without introducing any judgment or evaluation—to simply say what people are doing that we either like or don't like. Next, we state how we feel when we observe this action: are we hurt, scared, joyful, amused, irritated, etc? And thirdly, we say what needs of ours are connected to the feelings we have identified. An awareness of these three components is present when we use NVC to clearly and honestly express how we are.[3]

According to Rosenberg, we would be wise to do this to ensure compassion and understanding, but the second and equally imperative aspect is to get such information from the other person: What is she feeling and needing for enrichment? Again, I believe this is easier said than done, but it is a start that enhances our ability to see the value in others and perpetuate the spirit of this movement.

When having trouble seeing eye-to-eye with a fellow member of the movement, we can find common ground in the fact that, no matter what our experiences, we both may have a need to feel respected, validated, and appreciated. Focusing on those needs and how to create them for all involved may transcend current experiential conflict and maintain, if not strengthen, the spirit of the movement.

I recently heard Meganwind Eoyang, a leader in nonviolent communication, recite the following Edwin Markham poem, "Outwitted":

> He drew a circle that shut me out—
> Heretic, rebel, a thing to flout.
> But love and I had the wit to win.
> We drew a circle that took him in.[4]

Within the various experiences and outlooks that come with such an eclectic world, finding common ground is crucial. Markham's "love" and "wit to win" can provide major motivation for such things, but a practical component is imperative. The energy to create the strategies to work for Fat Acceptance is there, and those strategies have been created and executed. What is most interesting, and most telling, is that those strategies, like Markham's "wit to win," necessitates relationships, interdependence, and the recognition of both.

I do want to address my use and conflation of terms throughout the book. I know that Fat Activism, body positive activism, and Health At Every Size® activism are not interchangeable terms. Body positivism has been accused of taking focus off the bodies most maligned in Western society—fat bodies—which are the primary focus of Fat Activism. What's more, Health At Every Size® activism's focus on health and exercise do not sufficiently address the social, political, and aesthetic issues both Fat Activism and body positive activism address. These are just some of the differences between the movements. However, as will be discussed through the book, a strategic alignment of these movements—that is, looking at ways they intersect when thinking tactically about activism—may be in order, given the dictates of specific issues and situations. Thus, at times I will present these terms as working together, and consider body positivity and Health At Every Size® activism as tactical sub-categories or metonymies of Fat Acceptance.

This book is about observing the practical and tactical moves necessary to utilize the aforementioned zeitgeist to advance the understanding, acceptance, and respect—by self and others—that are the overarching goals of the Fat Acceptance movement. The ultimate goal, based on my assessment of Fat Activism and various other kinds of activism, is to alter hegemonic norms in ways that make room for the presence of fat people and the acknowledgment of misconceptions that have kept people of size in the margins of society.

Chapter 1, "Setting the Stage for Fat Activism," will introduce the movement, the common beliefs about correlations of weight and health, and the movement's major goal: to revise hegemonic takes on fat bodies. Through observation, one may glean an inadvertent overarching strategy akin to Anthony Giddens's concept of Structuration: the process in which an idea or ideology enters mainstream society through symbolism (Signification), institutions (Domination), and policy (Legitimation). This is the theory that will inform my observation of the tactics of fat activists.

Chapter 2, "Signification, Legitimation, and Domination in the Fat Acceptance Movement," elaborates on each aspect of Giddens's Structuration to show how specific aspects of the Fat Acceptance movement accomplish each with actions already established within activist circles. Thus, this is not a prescriptive take on Fat Activism, but an analysis of the rhetorical strategies already at play that work to rework meaning—of symbols, fat people, and human rights—to enhance the lives of fat people.

Chapter 3, "Fat Tactics and the Pragmatics of Fat Activism," moves away from the larger ideological motivations of Structuration to the more ground-level tactical work necessary to achieve success in Signfication, Domination, and Legitimation. The aforementioned interconnectedness promoted by nonviolent communication is framed as a pragmatic take on promoting acceptance and understanding through strategic moves. Using Jonathan Smucker's *Hegemony How-To: A Roadmap for Radicals* as a lens through which to interpret activists movements, I discern the immediate and localized need for narrative and pragmatic thought when taking the concrete step to achieve the real yet lofty goals of Structuration. At the risk of sounding prescriptive, I will discuss the partnership of pragmatism and agitation necessary to make activism affective while describing the ways in which Fat Activism, in particular, already accomplishes this.

Chapter 4, "Anti-fat Rhetoric and Social Media" explores how the Fat Acceptance movement works through a seemingly ubiquitous anti-fat rhetoric, significantly enhanced by social media, to accomplish its goals. The motivations of online trolls and cyberbullies are explored in an attempt to better understand one of the most difficult obstacles of Fat Acceptance at both individual and societal levels. This chapter serves as a kind of counterargument and refutation by analyzing the rhetoric of the movement's most vicious naysayers to discern true motivations that are not based in concerns for personal or societal health, but in creating and maintaining forms of hierarchy.

Chapter 5, "The Power of Narrative in Fat Acceptance," will harken back to the book's introduction, identify storytelling, on both a local and grand scale, as one of the most powerful and necessary tactics for activism. Returning to Smucker, I will explore the power of cocreating societal narratives and speculate as to how a purposefully malleable grand narrative of Fat Acceptance may look through Smucker's formulaic take on storytelling for political purposes. Thus, a particular rhetoric of storytelling—based on considerations of subject position and plot—is imperative.

The book's conclusion will reiterate a strain present throughout much of the book: the need to think pragmatically in activist movements. Considerations of Structuration, strategic activism, storytelling, and even dealing with anti-fat sentiment may do well to follow a practical plan that looks to change society as well as the esteem of fat activists. The success of the Fat Acceptance movement starts with the harnessing of the aforementioned zeitgeist, but may also include organized, pragmatic, and rhetorical considerations to reach its utmost effectiveness. This is not so much a prescription of what should happen, but a description of the many things that are happening *and working* within the movement.

NOTES

1. Diane F. Witmer, "The Construction of Self and Organization: Evoking Organizational Spirituality," *Essays on Communication and Spirituality*, ed. Amardo Rodriguez (New York: University Press of America, 2001), 7.
2. Ibid, 8.
3. Martin B. Rosenberg, *Nonviolent Communication: A Language of Life*, 2nd ed, (Encinitas, CA: Puddle Dancer Press, 2003), 8.
4. Edwin Markham, "Outwitted," accessed July 27, 2018, https://www.poetrynook.com/poem/outwitted.

Chapter One

Setting the Stage for Fat Activism

One may be hard-pressed to find an American, or, arguably, a citizen of Western civilization, who does not see a fat body as a negative that must be avoided. The nooks and crannies of society are full of signs that suggest as much: fat-free food, weight-loss programs, the confluence of the terms "fit" and "thin," the use of "fat" as a metonym for ignobility, weakness, ugliness, and other undesired states of being. One may even encounter some difficulty in finding those who may take issue with expressing one's disdain toward fat bodies. Charges for people to lose weight are often seen as battle cries for health and self-respect. Insulting a person of size is often construed as tough love, done for the fat person's own good. Indeed, anti-fat sentiment may be the last acceptable form of discrimination.

Why is anti-fat sentiment acceptable? We all know people who express disgust over fat bodies, deeming them inherently unattractive, and, by association, deeming those attracted to fat bodies as pathological or pathetic. Others see a fat body as a signpost for a severe lack of discipline, morality (fat people must indulge in the sin of gluttony, no?), and self-respect. Lastly, and, perhaps, most powerfully, fat is seen as unhealthy, a visual harbinger of disease and death. Although the initial reasons for anti-fat sentiment can be deemed a matter of taste, a concern for health—and a disdain for self-imposed ill health—is the major justification for such sentiment. The inherent unhealthiness of fat is a strong point if it is, indeed, categorically true.

However, an interdisciplinary cohort, existing of those in medicine, social science, and the humanities, have noticed flaws in both the science and logic of the antiobesity movement. Much of what society takes for granted as cause/effect relationship (fat = unhealthy) is, at best, inconclusive. Fat is correlated to illnesses like diabetes, but the causation has yet to be solidly proven. In fact, with the exception of osteoarthritis, caused by the pressure of increased body mass on joints, and "a few" cancers to which adipose tissue may contribute, causal links between fat and disease are still only hypothetical.[1] Linda Bacon, professor of nutrition and author of *Health at Every Size: The Surprising Truth about Your Weight*, explains that the reputation of fat as inherently unhealthy has been falsely presented as medical fact; this reputation has been "fueled by the power of money and cultural bias."[2] Based on sound, government-funded, scientific research, Bacon concludes that many public health officials, health advocates, and even scientists are complicit in supporting and promoting false information. She insists that a very different understanding of fat and health would emerge if we "suspend [our] preconceptions and open [our] hearts to scientific evidence."[3]

Paul Campos, author of *The Obesity Myth* has gone as far as calling obesity a faux disease. He writes, "The reason why the disease of obesity doesn't kill those who suffer from it and why it remains impossible to cure are one and the same: Because it doesn't exist."[4] Campos continues:

> "Obesity" is the name that medical science has given to that level of increasing body mass that, in and of itself, has significant negative consequences for a person's health. The problem with this definition is that, subject to exceptions at the extreme statistical margin, medical science has not been able to determine the existence of such a level, let alone fix its precise location. . . . Now that confounding variables such as activity levels are at last being taken into account, researchers have discovered that, except for the most extreme cases, the apparent relationship between body mass and health—which was weak to begin with—is in most instances random.[5]

Along with Campos and Bacon, organizations like the National Association to Advance Fat Acceptance (NAAFA) and the Association for Size Diversity and Health (ASDAH) work to expose the contradictory variables that weaken any claims to an obesity epidemic. ASDAH, an organization that abides by Bacon's Health At Every Size® (HAES®) ideology, provides a fact sheet listing studies that promote the difference between correlation and causation in scientific studies on fat and health. It reads, "There is considerable scientific evidence supporting the HAES® approach and establishing that 'obesity' is not the health risk it has been reported to be."[6]

Let's look at the actual terms. A mode of measurement like the body mass index (BMI) is, itself, flawed, deemed arbitrary, and insufficient, by scientists and medical professionals and does not truly take a diversity of body dynamics into account.[7] The connotations of the term "fat" are also important. In Fat Studies, terms like "overweight" and "obese," (the "O-words") hold far more negative connotations than the word "fat," which is seen as a mere descriptor, like "short" or "tall." To be "overweight" suggests the existence of a particular normal weight range that will always denote health and fitness. Such a range has yet to present itself. Thinness does not necessarily equate to health, and someone considered "overweight" can have a clean bill of health.[8] The "Obesity" connotations are far more destructive; they strongly suggest medical inferiority and disease.[9] (The terms "overweight" and "obesity" and its derivations will be placed in quotation marks throughout this work.)

These studies also expose the lack of efficacy in general dieting. Findings backed by Bacon, Campos, and many others prove that diets are often ineffective if not dangerous and counterproductive.[10] In "Prescription for Harm: Diet Industry Influence, Public Health Policy, and the 'Obesity Epidemic,'" Pat Lyons addresses the common misconceptions surrounding dieting and their neoliberal basis. Lyons writes that false or doctored (pardon the pun) medical information is presented to benefit the weight-loss industry.[11] Thus, Lyons writes a major point that not only echoes Bacon, Campos, and others who would expose the fallacious data of antiobesity, but exposes a salient point about the financial and aesthetic motivations behind fat stigma. "It is important to realize that were it not for weight bias, weight-loss programs would wither and die because they consistently fail to produce lasting weight loss. If concern for health is truly the primary motivation, then reducing fat stigma would be at the top of the list for health activism."[12]

Lyon's point drives my essay, "By Tort of Defamation: Anti-Fat Campaigns as Civil Wrongs toward People of Size." In this essay, I insist that anti-fat rhetoric is based on a very simple false syllogism:

> Being unhealthy is extremely detrimental to oneself and one's society.
> Fat is categorically and quintessentially unhealthy.
> Being fat is extremely detrimental to oneself and one's society.[13]

The fallacy can be found in the syllogism's first minor premise, "fat is categorically and quintessentially unhealthy." If data suggesting the inherent unhealthiness of fat is inconclusive, than the raison d'etre for antiobesity campaigns losses its power. Antiobesity becomes a movement of defamation based on aesthetic and neoliberal motivations.[14] This realization is where this book picks up. Anti-fat bias is not pro-health. It is something else. Once the medical claims given by those fighting a war on "obesity" are seen as weak or inconclusive, the war on fat is seen as prejudicial, discriminatory, unethical, and cruel.

Once the medical stigma of fat is deemed inconclusive or the animosity against fat and fat people has no moral backing—at that point—it becomes an issue of power. Like race, sex, and gender, fat becomes a tool for those who would like to express their superiority as well as those who would like to capitalize on that need for supremacy. From individuals looking for ways to squelch their own self-hatreds to corporations justifying their "get thin quick" schemes, fat is a tool of control and manipulation. Any inherent negativity given to fat is a fiction perpetuated by a narrative of control.

Of course, one can simply say that fat is not aesthetically pleasing and apply this to simple taste. That would be fine, if those who thought otherwise were not demonized for their preferences and ideas of beauty. The aesthetic argument (fat is simply unattractive; therefore, featuring fat bodies in fashion and various kinds of arts is simply bad taste and offensive behavior) is easily squelched by the idea of social construction and its relevance to beauty. Any marginalized group can tell you that their relation to beauty in a society is based on their relation to the beauty standards. Different races are, at best, exotically appealing, novel. Different sexualities are, at best, harbingers of comic relief, and fat bodies share a similar experience. At worst, however, these groups are offensive and considered a violent affront to staid sensibilities.

Unfortunately, the social construction of beauty as a theory can only go so far. If people of size will be accepted as beautiful and worthy of respect, they would do well to do one of two things: emulate the modes in which power is gained, the structures that need to be negotiated; or, destroy the structure, altogether. The all-out revolution necessary to accomplish the latter may not be ideal; Fat Activism is, after all, a movement to induce joy in life as well as fairness. However, a pragmatic approach to the former strategy may be a reasonable step in the right direction.

In "Making Room for Fat Studies in Writing Center Theory and Practice," I apply Harold Lasswell's formula for acquiring power in any given context. He renders this formula as follows:

> Man
> Pursues *Value*
> Through *Institutions*
> On *Resources*

When applying Fat Acceptance and Fat Studies to writing center contexts, the formula is rendered thusly,

> A Student
> Pursues *Enlightenment*
> Through *Academia*
> On Fat *Standpoint Epistemology*

In the context of a writing center (a place where students get guidance on their writing via face-to-face tutorials), both students and tutors of size would do well to use embodied ways of knowing—based on experiences as people of size—to further their learning and pedagogical approaches, respectively.[15]

I believe Lasswell's formula can work well for contexts larger than writing centers. Indeed, Lasswell's *Power and Personality* was written with larger contexts in mind. However, when the seeker of knowledge is a person of size, and the context is that of a fat-phobic American society, Lasswell's formula needs significant elaboration if we are to understand the situation well enough to speculate solutions.

As we clearly observed in the previous chapter, many relatively reasonable, often well-intentioned people become unpleasant when combatting Fat Acceptance, even when presented with well-researched information. Surely, civil forms of disagreement are deteriorating for reasons ranging from internet anonymity to subconscious emulation of daytime talk shows, but I believe the vitriol launched at Fat Acceptance may have deeper origins.

I believe this is an issue of Discourse. (I will use a capital "D" as does James Gee, whose definition of "Discourse" I will use throughout this work.) According to Gee,

> Discourses are ways of being in the world, or forms of life which integrate words, acts, values, beliefs, attitudes, social identities, as well as gestures, glances, body positions and clothes. . . . A Discourse is a sort of "identity kit" which comes complete with the appropriate costume and instructions on how to act, talk, and often write, so as to take on a particular role that others will recognize.[16]

A Discourse is an ideological—reflecting certain standpoints—and relatively exclusive source of cultural capital and power, but its resistance to "internal criticism and self-scrutiny" may be most relevant to our purposes. Gee explains that Discourse, itself, "defines what counts as acceptable criticism."[17] Typically, when two parties disagree, each is representing a particular ideology through a particular Discourse. Yes, they disagree, but each party recognizes the other party as an established Discourse worthy of argumentation. "But what one cannot do," explains Gee, "is stand outside all Discourses and criticize any one or all of them. Criticism must always be lodged from some set of assumed values, attitudes, beliefs and ways of talking/writing and, thus, from within some Discourse."[18]

Activists and supporters of Fat Acceptance and the Health At Every Size® ideology are traditionally deemed "outside all Discourse" according to traditional Discourses of virtue, health, and so forth. As Fat Acceptance activists know, pro-accepting and pro-fat Discourses exist but are not commonly recognized; they are invisible to most. Fat Acceptance and HAES® Discourses may overlap with other established Discourses (e.g. Feminism), but claims of fat being healthy, morally acceptable, beautiful, and so on constitute a completely foreign Discourse to most. Without a recognizable Discourse, a person's standpoint is not considered legitimate. There is no framework in which the ideas are housed. It is like entering a collegiate athletic tournament with no school affiliation and no official uniform. One may be very talented in that particular sport, but the tournament officials will not allow participation. Fat Acceptance has been locked out of the Discourse games.

Without a Discourse, one has no effective ethos. As many Fat Acceptance activists and Fat Studies scholars know, the Fat Acceptance movement, as well as body positivity and HAES® movements, have substantial logic behind their arguments, and the narratives presented by various scholars and authors within the movement provide heartfelt and empathetic stories of stigmatization and triumph over bigotry. Of course, the first and, arguably, most salient aspect of a Fat Acceptance Discourse is the interpretation of the term "fat." Like the term "queer" in LGBTQ communities, fat has been reclaimed by Fat Studies scholars and fat activists as anything from a mere descriptor to a synonym for beauty. Ultimately, any Fat Acceptance Discourse will revolve around the interpretations and reinterpretations of this term. In *Taking Up Space: How Eating Well and Exercising Regularly Changed My Life*, a book that works to bust myths that fat people do not take care of themselves or cannot be healthy, Pattie Thomas writes:

> In popular discourse, "fat" is a noun that describes the very essence of the fat. A person *is* unconditionally fat, and a fat person is unconditionally ugly, lazy, unhealthy, and disgusting.
>
> I have learned to regard fat as a description, a simple characteristic of the human body. Unfortunately, for me and for many people like me, the word "fat" comes with baggage. Fat Acceptance is about examining that baggage and asking new questions about generally accepted ideas. Fat Acceptance is about looking at the human body with different glasses. Fat Acceptance is about removing a stigma that hurts not only the stigmatized, but a stigma that hurts all humans.[19]

Of course, Gee's "acts, values, beliefs, attitudes, social identities," and so forth, also come into play. Activist Marilyn Wann has been building Gee's version of Discourse for the fat community for years. In the foreword to *The Fat Studies Reader*, Wann writes that self-reflexivity and the acknowledgment of one's subject position, including one's own intersectionality, is imperative to any activist and scholar within the movement.[20] By extension, she insists that an attempt to approach Fat Studies as objectively as possible may cause more harm than good: "Claims of neutrality or subjectivity in Fat Studies risk making analyses less credible, not more."[21] Thus, Fat Acceptance activism and Fat Studies rely heavily on narrative rhetoric, for example, autoethnography, and combine personal narrative with theoretical and scientific approaches. These are aspects of a burgeoning Discourse of Fat Acceptance.

A high level of defiance may also shape Fat Acceptance Discourse. Ragen Chastain, an activist and author for Fat Acceptance, has contributed heavily to this aspect of the Discourse. Her blog, *Dances with Fat*, chronicles her observations of society as a woman of size and exudes an attitude of speaking truth to power that tends to be the common tone of Fat Acceptance literature. Also, she consistently promotes the imperative to be absolutely unapologetic about one's body size. Her advice to would-be activists, scholars, and members of Fat Acceptance: "Stop negative body talk, including about your own body. That alone could start a revolution."[22] In her book *Fat: The Owner's Manual*, Chastain speaks of the need to "come out of the closet," as it were. Because one cannot effectively hide his or her body type, the metaphor isn't perfect. However, Chastain explains, "Obviously, there's no need for [fat people] to come out as fat, but there is another coming out that we can do. We can come out as fat *and* happy."[23] This is to say that Fat Acceptance Discourse is one that does not reflect society's mandate that all fat people feel shame for their fat. Being happy while fat inherently counters fat bias and is a major aspect of Fat Acceptance Discourse.

The physical, sartorial, and generally aesthetic implications of Gee's Discourse also come into play and will be addressed thoroughly in this book. For now, one can glean from the above references that a Discourse of Fat Acceptance is alive and growing. However, this Discourse's recognition in mainstream society will take more than strong-willed activists, scholars, and writers. References to both quantitative and qualitative data, scientific and ethnographic findings, seem difficult to process for many. The Fat Acceptance movement and the academic field of Fat Studies still lack hegemonic ethos to mainstream society. In fact, those with anti-fat sentiments and ideologies do not seem to acknowledge the logical and emotional appeals inherent in Fat Acceptance Discourse because the perceived lack of ethos is both blinding and deafening.

Rhetoricians refer to ethos as credibility of one's character or one's "ethical" right to speak on a subject. According to Aristotle—and, to an extent, common sense—we tend to believe "fair-minded" people more deeply and easily than others.[24] Of course, "fair-minded" is a description contingent on an audience. "Fair-mindedness," then, is reflected through one's choice of words, one's style, one's overall Discourse. Basically, if we don't sound like our audience, or sound like people our audience respects, we won't be nearly as persuasive as we would like to be, if at all. No Discourse, no ethos. No ethos, no respect.

How we sound goes a long way, for ethos is not just about professional credibility—which does count for something—but on-the-spot rhetorical savvy. In situations where "there is not exact knowledge but room for doubt" credibility "should result from the speech, not from a previous opinion that the speaker is a certain kind of person."[25] This is why references to scientific studies and well-researched texts about weight/health correlations often fall on deaf ears. This is why authorities like Paul Campos and Linda Bacon can be dismissed by commenters that have never set eyes on a text about size and health. This is why activists like Ragen Chastain are bombarded by blog comments refuting her viewpoint and, therefore, her very existence.

What can be done? Initially, we can continue to do what we do. There is already a Discourse to Fat Acceptance, to be sure, but it is just beginning to break into social consciousness. Fat Activists are appearing on talk shows, news segments, and televised debates; this is a good thing. Plus-size models are beginning to break into the fashion industry—also a good thing. I wonder, though, if meta-knowledge about what we do can quicken and strengthen the process. If we see the social construction of Fat Acceptance Discourse as a structure in which the already rousing spirit of this movement can be enhanced, would it more quickly break the horizon of social consciousness?

Lasswell's aforementioned formula for acquiring power is, itself, powerful in its simplicity, but we get a more thorough blueprint from Anthony Giddens's Structuration theory. In *The Constitution of Society: Outline of the Theory of Structuration*, Giddens breaks down the ways in which Discourses are created: (1) Signification (symbolic action; language); (2) Legitimation (normative action); and (3) Domination (allocation or authorization of resources).[26] I am interested in exploring each structure and its potential benefits to bolstering the Fat Acceptance Movement and helping its concomitant Discourse come into societal light. To be clear, actual creation of the Discourse is unnecessary; it is already alive and well. However, maybe looking at Fat Acceptance through the lenses of Giddens's three structures can create a brighter spotlight for it.[27]

The first of Giddens's three "structural dimensions of social systems" is Signification. By Signification, Giddens means the way people interact with society through communicative practices: language, signs, images, and so forth. Each aforementioned "identity kit" has distinct communicative practices—although they may overlap with other practices in other Discourses—that popularize, perpetuate, and strengthen the values of the Discourse. According to Giddens's Signification, certain signs and symbols are expected and others aren't. In fact, the symbols that aren't are either dismissed outright or "transmuted"—made sense of—as something quirky, odd, situational, and so forth.

For example, a symbol like the Venus of Willendorf, an ancient figurine of a fat, feminine body that apparently dates back to 24,000 BCE, may represent the beauty of the fat female body within Fat Acceptance circles, but is "made sense of" outside such circles as an aesthetic of a primitive, less civilized culture. So, instead of seeing the figure as a version of beauty, it is deemed a mistaken take on beauty by a less evolved society. In fact, the figure was called "Venus" out of sarcasm when initially discovered in the nineteenth century.[28]

So, how does one start to project images of beautiful and handsome fat bodies into the mainstream? People are definitely going for it. Substantia

Jones's *Adipositivity Project* is one way, although that, too, has been mocked by pop culture figures like Daniel Tosh.[29] Other mainstream symbols are being appropriated by Fat Acceptance, like the reclining female silhouette on so many tractor trailer mudflaps and Wonder Woman (my favorite). These are examples of visual activism, even if the creators of the images didn't intend it.

As we have already seen, terminology is a key aspect to Discourse. The reclaiming of the word "fat" as a simple descriptor and an adjective that, for many in the Fat Acceptance movement, has connotations of aesthetic appeal, has been key. Also, I've noticed the language of fat admirers expressing the idea that the fat body is a more natural, earthly and "real" body. Although the danger of flipping discrimination around to shame thin bodies is too great for my tastes, one should not ignore the ways people are talking about fat bodies, taking words with societally-accepted positive connotations—abundance, fullness, natural—and applying them to fat bodies. Maybe more of this needs to happen.

Paul Delacroix, in *Abundance* magazine, passionately writes about fat female bodies in a tone indicative of new romantic poetry and prose: "I only know what I consider beautiful. I love mountains and seashores with white sandy beaches, and I love flowers in full bloom instead of tight, compressed budding ones . . . and I love grain fields full of bounty, and trees heavy with fruit. I love nature and growth. And I love fat women."[30] People may not want to wax poetic with every chance they have to discuss Fat Acceptance, but the attitude that feels such appreciation for fat bodies should not be entirely squelched to satisfy societal expectations. Let such appreciation pepper our prose by manifesting in adjectives and adverbs that connote fat positivity.

Of course, none of this may effectively squelch those who strictly correlate weight and health. These people will say that fat is categorically unhealthy and will lead to grave illness or premature death. Thus, fat athletes are imperative symbols of Fat Acceptance. The article, "Olympians. . . . They Come in All Shapes and Sizes" in the Fat Acceptance blog *Fierce, Freethinking Fatties* provides several images that may need further perpetuation.[31] HAES® ideology is a concept that needs to be *seen* just as much as it needs to be *heard*. Lastly, Chastain (an athlete, herself) and her concept of "fat and happy" come into play: a fat person who walks with swagger, wears a smile on her face and isn't the picture of illness, depression, and self-loathing that fat-phobic society expects; an ally spreading the word about HAES® ideology and civil rights for people of all size.

The signification of Fat Acceptance comes in the language we use and the images we create—images that are both original creations and appropriations of popular symbols. This is not the whole story, but it's a great place to start.

Within his theory, Giddens considers "Legitimation," the next structural dimension of social systems, as the "theory of normative regulation" actualized by legal institutions. The Fat Acceptance movement is well aware of the importance of normalizing the fat body from a legal perspective. NAAFA, the National Association to Advance Fat Acceptance, sites civil rights as one of its main reasons for existing. Of course, the difficulty fat people have had regarding size discrimination is nothing new within the movement. Working around this trend has been both tricky and painful, even for the success stories. Although old news for many, some may not be aware of the current legal climate for those suffering from anti-fat bias and workplace discrimination; they do not realize that, according to the law, fat people are not "legitimate." Fortunately, a few places already recognize the need to protect people from weight discrimination. According to NAAFA.org, the state of Michigan and the cities of Washington, DC; Santa Cruz; San Francisco; Binghamton, New York; Urbana, Illinois; and Madison, Wisconsin, already have laws in place to protect fat people.[32] Outside of these places, however, fat people and those who represent them must actually cater to the fat-shaming ideologies systemic throughout many institutions, including workplaces and courtrooms. According to attorneys Dylan Vade and Sondra Solovay, the only way to win lawsuits against fat discrimination is to admit that there is, indeed, something wrong with being fat. They write of Toni and John, two people who sued former employers for weight-based dismissal. Toni lost her case, but John won over $1,000,000. Before attributing each person's result to his and her respective lawyers, consider the importance of each plaintiff's attitude:

> Both Toni and John encountered discrimination. Toni refused to locate the problem in, or on, her body, finding instead that the obstacle was the fat-phobic attitudes she faced (Cassista, 1999). Rejecting a medicalized view, she argued that she was perceived as disabled because of her weight, but that there was nothing "medically wrong" with her. Her argument is noteworthy because there were no apologies and nothing repentant in her tone.
>
> John's approach was that his weight constituted a physiological disorder. He agreed that there was a problem with his body, that something was "wrong." He had tried fasting, hypnosis, and even having his jaws wired shut in his attempts to become a thin person.Toni was fiercely proud. She lost her case. John was apologetic. He won.[33]

One can glean from Giddens that Legitimation is the normalization of a status, behavior, lifestyle, or belief by formal policy. John's legal win is not Legitimation, for his fat body was not normalized but seen as a bad thing he was not given an adequate chance to overcome.

Some victims of fat discrimination have fallen back on disability law without feeling like they necessarily have a disability. Referencing and using disability laws are their only option. The Equal Employment Opportunity Commission recently won a case for Ronald Kratz, a worker for a military vehicle manufacturer, by claiming his fat as a disability. Whether Kratz feels disabled or not isn't clear. He was qualified to do his job, according to an article in the *Houston Chronicle*, but his employer's neglect to offer him accommodations for his "disability" won him a modest compensation. Kratz was not offered his old job or another job within the company. He may have won, but he is not legitimate.[34] I cannot imagine fighting workplace discrimination by using the idea that African-Americans are inferior: "Your honor, it's not my client's fault he couldn't do the job. He's black. Instead of firing him, his employer should have given him a more menial position. If there's no position available, my client should be financially compensated." That, too, would not be legitimation.

So, what can be done about this? First of all, Giddens's structural dimensions substantially overlap. Thus, we may do well to connect fat with other normalized entities or beliefs (connecting Fat Acceptance with Women's Studies or recognizing Fat Acceptance as a diversity issue), reappropriate terms like "fat," and make people aware of the nonconclusive science behind the medicalization of fat—all things currently being done. What's more, showing people the legal precedents already set in various cities and the entire state of Michigan will show that the normalization process has already begun. Even if people stigmatize fat bodies in general, they may still support laws protecting employees and patients with fat bodies, as a study by the Rudd Center suggests.[35]

I think seeking Legitimation is a necessary move, especially when protecting employees as well as patients and students. However, we need not wait for the law to tell us that fat bodies are legitimate bodies. We must keep on normalizing fat within our own lives, exemplify this normalization, and know (and show) that fat people are worthy of admiration and respect.

Lastly, Giddens defines Domination as a structural feature of society and an inherent aspect of social interaction.[36] My use of Giddens's term here does not come as an invitation to dominate anyone or anything; it is a call to recognize and understand Dominance in order to help accomplish the mission of Fat Acceptance.

So what and where is Dominance? Giddens's Dominance comes in two forms: Allocative (Domination over objects) and Authoritative (Dominance over people). Where Allocation is more aligned with economic institutions, Authority is more aligned with the political.[37] I think for our purposes—the empowerment and exposition of Fat Acceptance—we can combine these two things. Since there is no shortage of tried and true Discourses that reflect political and economic institutions, we may do well to notice where Fat

Acceptance overlaps with them. The point is not to have Fat Acceptance usurped by other institutions, but to see those institutions as possible platforms on which Fat Acceptance can build its own.

Thus, acknowledging and working with intersections are key. I see this done most affectively with Fat Studies, an emerging field in academia, where Allocative and Authoritative Dominance are apparent. In an essay titled "Teaching Fat Studies: From Conception to Reception," Patti Watkins and Amy Farrell recognize that each Fat Studies syllabus they examined contained an articulation of intersectionality, if not an identification of intersectionality as a distinct course goal. One syllabus explicitly wanted students to develop an ability to "Describe how body weight is an area of human difference subject to privilege and discrimination that intersects with other systems of oppression in the U.S. based on gender, race, class, age, sexual orientation, and ability."[38] Even when met with resistance by students who did not see the relevance of Fat Studies, let alone its connections to other affinity groups, Watkins cited her university's established mission statement and policy on diversity.[39] Connecting Fat Studies to preestablished and respected fields while also connecting to established university policy is a good example of noticing structures of Dominance and working *with* them.

According to both Watkins and Farrell, there is significant buy-in for Fat Studies courses because of both genuine interest among students and the overlapping interests of other programs and disciplines.[40] Malcolm Gladwell speaks to this in his book *The Tipping Point*, when he writes of the importance of mavens, connectors, and the concept of "stickiness" in changing paradigms. The mavens (atypically knowledgeable people) and connectors (people who bring different parties with similar interests together) can create stickiness (the ability to keep people interested).[41] By analogy, academics (both mavens and connectors) create stickiness (popularity and respect) through seeing Fat Studies (and, by association, Fat Acceptance) as a systemic aspect of academia. One can find an appropriate place for it in many disciplines (sociology, law, English, art history, communications, health sciences, healthcare, social work, cultural studies, multi-cultural studies, women's and gender studies, psychology, etc.). Working with these potentialities can and does strengthen Fat Studies.

We would do well to find the social analogy to Fat Studies's success. Where does Fat Acceptance overlap with tried and true paradigms? Giddens's concept of Signification can speak to this (all structures of social systems overlap). The appropriation of pop cultural icons, for example, Wonder Woman, by those in the Fat Acceptance movement can go a long way, but the reclamation of the term "fat" as either a neutral descriptor or positive adjective—many have appropriated the term "phat" from hip hop parlance—may be very important.

The idea that definition is a foundational concept to any attempt to persuade goes as far back as Plato and Socrates.[42] Taking back the word fat, like the LGBTQ community's embrace of "queer," is a powerful political move. It not only provides esteem and enthusiasm among fat people, but plants a seed in the collective conscious of society. Such a seed may sprout into a necessary thought: the words "fat" and "pride" can go hand in hand.

In addition, the intersectionality of other body-centered activists groups could help. As I mention in the book's introduction, Body Positivity and HAES® ideology are not synonyms with Fat Acceptance, but the overlap of all three movements is clear in the general message that the demonization of fat bodies will not be tolerated. At times—time being more kairotic (situational) than chronological—embracing the overlaps more than the differences may come in handy when gauging which movement may have the Allocative or Authoritarian dominance at a specific time. This tactical move is not an erasure of each movement's distinctions; it is a way to use Giddens's Dominance as strategically as possible.

So, we start to see a general plan for Fat Acceptance activism. Although we can use certain established structures of society to bolster Fat Acceptance, we can also level the playing field by identifying the structures that perform fat bias and, ourselves, engage in nonviolent protest. If about 70 percent of the American population is fat, a boycott from this demographic cannot be good for any corporation's bottom line (I'm thinking airlines, companies that use images of fat people in negative ways, etc.). In all of this, people must be (a) equipped with facts and (b) equipped to present those facts within the confines of a variety of Discourses. That is, academia respects a specific kind of presentation, and corporate America respects another. Misinterpreting the rhetorical situation can do more harm than good, even if one's facts are solid. The main point is that people are the ones that give established institutions their power; they have a say in how these institutions conduct themselves and operate.

If we recognize how power is enacted and how we can possibly relate to those enactments, we can change things. In *Power and Personality*, Harold Lasswell provides a model for how people acquire power: people pursue specific values through institutions based on the resources they have to offer. Fat activists can both contribute to aspects of established institutions (academia, for example) or threaten the viability of established institutions by hitting them in the wallet, for example. To recognize Dominance in society is to recognize power—who has it and how to acquire it.

The following chapter will give more thorough attention to each of Giddens structures.

NOTES

1. Paul Campos, Abigail Saguy, Paul Ernsberger, Eric Oliver, Glenn Gaesser, "The Epidemiology of Overweight and Obesity: Public Health Crisis or Moral Panic?" *International Journal of Epidemiology*, 35 (2006): 57.
2. Linda Bacon, *Health at Every Size: The Surprising Truth about Your Weight* (Dallas: Benbella Books, 2010), Kindle edition, ch. 6.
3. Ibid.
4. Paul Campos, *The Obesity Myth: Why America's Obsession with Weight is Hazardous to Your Health* (New York: Gotham Books, 2004), 42.
5. Ibid.
6. "Health at Every Size® Fact Sheet," Association for Size Diversity and Health (2011), https://www.sizediversityandhealth.org/content.asp?id=161.
7. Campos, *The Obesity Myth,* xxiii.
8. Campos, *The Obesity Myth,* xxiii.
9. Dylan Vade and Sondra Solovay, "No Apology: Shared Struggle in Fat and Transgender Law," *The Fat Studies Reader*, ed. Esther Rothblum and Sondra Solovay (New York: New York University Press, 2009), 167–175.
10. "Health at Every Size® Fact Sheet," Association for Size Diversity and Health (2011), https://www.sizediversityandhealth.org/content.asp?id=161.
11. Pat Lyons, "Prescription for Harm: Diet Industry Influence, Public Health Policy, and the 'Obesity Epidemic,'" *The Fat Studies Reader*, ed. Esther Rothblum and Sondra Solovay (New York: New York University Press, 2009), 78–85.
12. Ibid.
13. Ibid.
14. Erec Smith, "By Tort of Defamation: Anti-Fat Campaigns as Civil Wrongs toward People of Size," *Issues: Understanding Controversy and Society* (ABC-CLIO, 2014. Accessed 17 Sept. 2014), 7.
15. Erec Smith, "Making Room for Fat Studies in Writing Center Theory and Practice" *Praxis: A Writing Center Journal*. Winter 2013. Accessed 15 March 2016.
16. James Gee, *Social Linguistics and Literacies: Ideology in Discourse*. (London: Falmer Press, 1990), 142.
17. Ibid.
18. Ibid., 144.
19. Pattie Thomas, *Taking Up Space: How Eating Well and Exercising Regularly Changed My Life* (Nashville, TN: Pearlsong Press, 2005), Kindle edition, Loc 443–452.
20. Marilyn Wann, Foreword to *The Fat Studies Reader*, ed. Esther Rothblum and Sondra Solovay. 1st ed. (New York: New York University Press, 2009), xiii.
21. Ibid., xviii.
22. Ragen Chastain, "A Very Good Place to Start," *Dances with Fat* (blog), June 8, 2015, https://danceswithfat.wordpress.com/2015/06/08/a-very-good-place-to-start/
23. Ragen Chastain, *Fat: The Owner's Manual* (Austin, TX: Sized for Success, 2012), 180.
24. Aristotle, *On Rhetoric*, trans. by George A. Kennedy (New York: Oxford University Press, 2007), 38.
25. Ibid., 38–39.
26. Anthony Giddens, *The Constitution of Society: Outline of the Theory of Structuration*, (Berkeley: University of California Press, 1984).
27. I know that Gee and Giddens use different definitions of discourse and ideology, but more important here is the construction and perpetuation of a world view. I believe Giddens's structural dimensions can help us understand the construction of Gee's Discourse.
28. Christopher Witcombe, "Venus of Willendorf," *Art History Resources*, 2005, http://arthistoryresources.net/willendorf/.
29. In 2010, the comedian Daniel Tosh took a body-positive photo from Substantia Jones's Adipositivity Project and poked fun at it on his television show *Tosh.0*. The uproar from the Fat Acceptance community caused Tosh to take the photo down soon afterwards.

30. Paul Delacroix, "Why I Find Supersized Women Beautiful," *BBW_Art.* May 24, 2016, https://bbwart.wordpress.com/paul-delacroix/.

31. Erilyn, "Olympians. . . . They Come In All Shapes and Sizes," *Fierce, Freethinking Fatties.* Aug 3, 2012, https://fiercefatties.com/2012/08/03/olympians-they-come-in-all-shapes-and-sizes/.

32. "Weight Discrimination Laws," 2016, http://www.naafaonline.com/dev2/education/laws.html.

33. Dylan Vade and Sondra Solovay, "No Apology: Shared Struggles in Fat and Transgender Law," *The Fat Studies Reader*, ed. Esther Rothblum and Sondra Solovay, 1st ed (New York: NYU Press, 2009), 168.

34. L. M. Sixel, "Fired Obese Worker Will Get $55,000," *The Houston Chronicle,* July 24, 2012, http://www.chron.com/business/article/Fired-obese-worker-will-get-55-000-3732044.php.

35. Amanda Cuda, "Yale Study: Citizens Support Ban of Weight-based Discrimination," *Connecticut Post*, June 27 2010, http://www.ctpost.com/news/article/Yale-study-Citizens-support-ban-of-weight-based-538429.php.

36. Giddens, 32.

37. Ibid., 33.

38. Patti Lou Watkins, Amy Farrell, and Andrea Doyle Hugmeyer, "Teaching Fat Studies: From Conception to Reception," Oregon State University, April 27, 2012, http://oregonstate.edu/instruct/pp/ctla-files/docs/teaching-fat-studies.pdf, 9.

39. Ibid.

40. Ibid.

41. Malcolm Gladwell, *The Tipping Point: How Little Things Can Make a Big Difference* (New York: Back Bay Books, 2002).

42. In the closing section of *Phaedrus*, Socrates says this about the importance of definition and knowing one's audience (a point I make later in this post): "Until a man knows the truth of the several particulars of which he is writing or speaking, and is able to define them as they are, and having defined them again to divide them until they can be no longer divided, and until in like manner he is able to discern the nature of the soul, and discover the different modes of discourse which are adapted to different natures, and to arrange and dispose them in such a way that the simple form of speech may be addressed to the simpler nature, and the complex and composite to the more complex nature—until he has accomplished all this, he will be unable to handle arguments according to rules of art, as far as their nature allows them to be subjected to art, either for the purpose of teaching or persuading—such is the view which is implied in the whole preceding argument."

Chapter Two

Signification, Legitimation, and Domination in the Fat Acceptance Movement

SIGNIFICATION IN THE FAT ACCEPTANCE MOVEMENT

Signification, especially for our purposes, will focus on the symbols that promote Fat Acceptance as well as a reimagining of symbols that have been either neutral (regarding Fat Acceptance) or anti-fat. Because visual rhetoric is a primary medium for many people, the importance of image signification is clear. However, signification also refers to the use of terms. Like symbols, these terms range from words that were initially neutral to those that were initially anti-fat. "Signifieds" have been swapped to promote both activism and the constructed nature of attitudes and ideologies solidified by repetition and institutional backing instead of essential, ontological truth. Thus, the importance of Signification is two-fold: it promotes Fat Acceptance in expedient ways while also exposing the arbitrary nature of meaning making, generally.

Activism as signification may be the most aesthetically-based aspect of the Fat Acceptance movement for obvious reasons. However, words and concepts do not escape this strategy's purview. Familiar words have been given unfamiliar, fat positive meanings. Also, new words have been coined as clever and powerful plays on more common words.

As we already know, the term "fat" has lost its negative connotations within the Fat Acceptance movement. At the very least, it is a neutral term denoting a bodily description and nothing more. It's less than positive cousin, "obese," on the other hand, has been abandoned as too negative and medicalized to appropriate for fat activists' purposes. Beyond being a mere descriptor, "fat" has been synthesized with other aspects of fat activist signification to empower Fat Acceptance. The term "fatshion," for example, synthesizes the words "fat" and "fashion" to give a fat positive label to the Fat Acceptance movement's foray into fashion and beauty industries. "Fatshionistas" can be found throughout the internet and fashion magazines. Their success has already inspired major household names in American culture, for example, the magazine *Sports Illustrated*[1] and the retailer JC Penney.[2]

Words are surely an important part of Fat Activists' forays into Signification. Regarding Fat Acceptance, Margo Demello identifies some key terms, including "Fat Shaming," "Headless Fatties" (the inevitable video of fat bodies in public, shot only from the neck down, when television media discusses the obesity epidemic), "Chubby Chasers" (gay men who are sexually attracted to fat men), "thinspiration" (inspirational images or speech that promote the acquisition of thinness), "folk devil" (another term for scapegoat that, in this context, denotes fat people as a societal scourge).[3]

As will be seen, images and maxims can be gamed or fitted with altered content to promote an alternative message in ways indicative of well-accepted images and maxims. Health professional and fat activist, Kelly Bliss, teaches size-acceptance exercise classes under the logo "Lifestyle Watchers"—a clear play on Weight Watchers. "Lifestyle Watchers" provides a community of people who know that size does not necessarily determine the presence or absence of health, a thought modeled by the symbols of three people of small, medium, and large build, respectively, in the logo (figure 2.1). Bliss states, "It is my intention, in the future, to use the well-known reputation of weight watchers to slingshot lifestyle watchers and the body acceptance movement into the mainstream."[4]

Words and a general Discourse of Fat Acceptance, which I will address more thoroughly in chapter 5, are integral in changing ideas about fat people. However, Signification is a largely visual mode of Giddens Structuration, as

Figure 2.1. Lifestyle Watchers Logo, http://www.kellybliss.com/main/index.php Used by permission.

well. In fact, much visual representation in Fat Activism results from the purposeful reappropriation of well-known images to support Fat Acceptance. Placing a new signifier into an accepted signified is one way to create a fat-positive sign. Ragen Chastain, upon looking at an inspirational poem in a gym, has her own experience with this.

> I also like to "recreate" memes that are created with fat bodies but questionable messages that are often seen as positive but aren't when further examined. For example, recently there was a picture of a fat person on a piece of gym equipment (taken from behind) with the message "Make fun of a fat person at the gym is like making fun of a homeless person at a job fair." I changed it to read "Making fun of a fat person or a homeless person is a shitty thing to do no matter where they are. Don't be an asshole."[5]

Chastain's general thoughts also apply to altering a signifier to be clearly different but still contain enough traditional traits to remain recognizable. This means letting fat people dwell in spaces from which they are typically barred. She writes,

> I think that one of the most powerful things we can do is to show fat bodies, whether they are performing athletic feats or doing dishes. Fat people face a massive lack of positive representation in all aspects of the media. When we do see ourselves it's typically without a head—as a cautionary tale, or a before picture in a diet ad. We are told directly and indirectly that fat bodies aren't fit to be seen, let alone loved, and so showing images of happy fat people is a critical way to push back against that and to give other fat people a chance to see people who look like them and are happy with their bodies.[6]

As an example, placing a fat body in contexts traditionally owned by thin ones, let us explore one of the most prominent symbols in the Fat Acceptance movement: the reimagining of female super heroes as fat women. Although other powerful symbols of Fat Acceptance do exist, the depiction of Wonder Woman with a fat body may be very relevant at the moment. This is a time when the rebirth of Woman Wonder as a popular figure and her introduction into cinema coincides with the rise of Fat Acceptance. Thus, utilizing the symbol of a powerful female superhero to represent a traditionally powerless female demographic can be quite powerful, especially to women of size who have never imagined the inherent power of those with their body types. Fat Wonder Woman has been seen in various spaces of Fat Acceptance. At the 2012 conference for NAAFA, images of fat Wonder Woman were passed out to conference goers. The internet is full of images—non-sarcastic—of fat wonder women, either as drawings or photographs of fat women in the hero's garb.

Fat Wonder Women

Analyzing the impetus behind the choice of Wonder Woman as a prominent fat activist revision may give some insight into the importance of signification within the movement. First, an anecdote. Two years ago, a few friends and I decided to have a Halloween party at a local pub. Most friends showed up in something homemade or something that didn't take much care or thought. (At one point, I expected to see someone wearing a white sheet with two eye holes cut into it.) I had my old standby, a Jedi outfit with light saber accessory. (I guess I had to be Mace Windu.) Just when I began to think that I was the only person who put an iota of thought into his costume, the sight of a good friend changed my mind. My friend is a very large woman—big and tall—and, in my opinion, one of the most gorgeous women in town. She wore a full, professional-grade Wonder Woman outfit. She looked spectacular. In a fat-hating culture like ours, wearing such a costume was a definite risk to my friend's social and emotional well-being. She was strong and secure enough—a Wonder Woman in her own right—to express herself as such a woman, outright. I was in awe of her beauty and strength. And that is what Wonder Woman is: beauty and strength.

Weeks later, I discovered a website that focused exclusively on drawings of Wonder Woman with a fat body. *The Big Beautiful Wonder Woman Blog* is the brainchild of Jamar Nicholas and was created simply to celebrate the image of a super woman of size while exploring our ideas of beauty. He writes, "I do this to see great artists go into this assignment with one rule: Create your version of a Big Beautiful Wonder Woman. Or flip it: Fat Wonder Woman. Is fat beautiful? Isn't it? That's for the artist to determine—not mine. I love to see what you come up with."[7] Although not an explicit goal of Nicholas, this site points to the potential power of Wonder Woman as that aforementioned icon of Fat Acceptance.

Despite the inadvertently political effects of Nicholas's blog, Wonder Woman is no stranger to political representation. Since gracing the cover of *Ms. Magazine* in the 1970s,[8] she has symbolized feminine strength in ways understandable to both men and women. However, in our current period of third-wave eclecticism, Wonder Woman has been rebooted into a powerful big, beautiful woman. Perhaps this quote from Wonder Woman's creator, William Moulton Marsten, is telling enough: "Frankly, Wonder Woman is psychological propaganda for the new type of woman who should, I believe, rule the world."[9]

Symbolizing beauty and strength throughout the Fat Acceptance Movement is not all Wonder Woman has to offer. Her specific skills provide a sufficient analogy for fighting fat stigmatization. Her general strength is clear enough. In order to do battle with anti-fat discrimination, especially the kind disguised as beneficence, and concern for either individual or societal health, one must have a strength of character unknown to more privileged and less stigmatized people. Her more specific tools, however, may give further insight into Wonder Woman's significance in the Fat Acceptance Movement.

Wonder Woman seems to represent survival as a symbol of Fat Acceptance; the slings and arrows of anti-fat sentiment must be deflected. Wonder Woman has bracelets strong enough to deflect bullets. Many in the Fat Acceptance Movement give warnings about insulting rhetoric when referring readers to a particular website or article bent on heralding the detriments of fat. These trigger warnings are common ways to alert people to a text's potential to offend, depress, or infuriate. (Ragen Chastain is excellent at providing such warnings throughout her *Dances with Fat* blog.) Being prepared for the onslaught of negativity is important; weathering the storm of anti-fat rhetoric and propaganda is a necessary tool for doing this work. One's ability to deflect must be quite strong. The "Stereotype Management Skills"[10] website created by the *Health At Every Size*® ideology may be a metaphorical bulletproof bracelet; it provides ways of deflecting fat stigma, specifically the stigma echoed and produced by HBO's 2012 *Weight of the Nation* documentary.[11]

Wonder Woman's insistence on truth is a very famous aspect of her character—if not the most famous. Wonder Woman's Lasso of Truth forces honesty and objectivity from anyone confined by it. Those in Fat Acceptance and Fat Studies often find themselves combating erroneous views about the correlations between weight and health. I see a metaphorical Lasso of Truth in the work of activists/scholars like Linda Bacon, Paul Campos, and Pattie Thomas, just to give a short list. These writers challenge the weight loss and pharmaceutical industries, insisting they finally tell the truth about weight and health. The aforementioned *Health At Every Size*® blog, along with the National Association to Advance Fat Acceptance and the Association for Size Diversity and Health could be seen as potential Lassos of Truth, as well. Those spreading anti-fat rhetoric may have their fallacious reasoning exposed by information provided by these sites. (Ragen Chastain writes about the spirit of championing the truth in the post "Everybody Galileo Now," in which she coins the term "Galileos": those who stand by the truth despite being bombarded with accepted but fallacious ideas.)[12]

All this is to say that Wonder Woman seems to work for the Fat Acceptance Movement. Using Big Beautiful Wonder Woman as a symbol of fat, female pride across race, sexuality, and socioeconomic status has been well embraced. Comic book creators, Suzan Colon and Jennifer Traig, echo this in their book, *What Would Wonder Woman Do?* This book is meant to give solid advice to working women. When giving advice about dealing with difficult people, the authors' advice is simple: be superior to them in every way, because your enemies "can't argue with the truth."[13] Not everyone knows the truth about weight and health and not everyone knows the truth about arbitrary and socially constructed standards of beauty. Fortunately, the Fat Acceptance Movement's appropriation of a beloved figure proves to be a powerful medium for these ideas.

Fatshion and Fatshionistas!

Adipositivity, a portmanteau of the words "adipose" (fat) and "positivity," is the name of another source of powerful Fat Acceptance symbolism. Substantia Jone's Adipositivity.com features several "regular" people of size in photographs emphasizing both beauty and sexuality to promote the idea that fat people, too, can embody such things. The site features non-professional models, alone, in a couple, or part of a group, posing for both pride for themselves and defiance of society's status quo for beauty and sexuality.[14]

Of course, the Adipositivity Project is meant to play with a tried and true pop genre: the pin-up model. Often bordering on what others may consider lewd and pornographic, Jone's project pushes the boundaries of expectation. A woman commonly deemed obese posing, naked, in satin sheets calls forth familiar images of female sexuality portrayed by an unfamiliar agent. A sparsely clad woman of size in a suggestive position cracks the lens through which our society views beauty, but in a way so familiar that initial dissonance transforms to curious exploration. What do we see when we see a bare-chested woman in a loving embrace with her thin lover? Something familiar yet new, curious, and intriguing.

When asked what images of the Fat Acceptance movement she found most useful or powerful, Jones had this to say:

> I'm careful to avoid some of the more sexualizing tropes of beauty and fashion photography. I'll never ask a model to arch her back or give the camera a come-hither. But there are many fashion/beauty poses I get a kick out of subverting. Not long ago I did a milk bath shot. We've seen them often. Face and limbs emerging from the surface. Sometimes breasts. But where's the belly? Mine allowed the Adiposer's belly to form a plump, round island in the tub of milk. Well, non-dairy creamer, actually.
>
> I think the Fat Acceptance images I find to be the most effective are the ones which say to the viewer, "I am confident. I am powerful. I am *you*."[15]

Jones's project has not gone without ridicule. To many, the thought of a fat, naked body does not challenge beauty norms or create a mind-altering dissonance. The sight of a fat woman performing confident sexuality has induced laughter in the same ways that D. Diane Davis may call a break in totality. The popular comedian Daniel Tosh usurped one of Jone's photos, a picture of model Janie Martinez hailing a cab while topless, and used it for a very popular segment of his hit television show, *Tosh.0*.[16] The picture was on the show's website until complaints from fat activists flooded the site. The picture was eventually taken down, but the message had been loud and clear: your celebration of sexual pride does not belong in this society in any way other than a crass joke.

Fashion model, photographer, and editor, Velvet D'Amour, presents herself and others with fat bodies as prominent sex symbols. Her magazine, *Volup2* features models who are typically deemed unattractive—often because of fat bodies—by mainstream society. D'Amour, a fat person herself, writes,

> I suppose some of my strength lies in taking what may be seen as average, if not "unattractive," and bringing out the beauty that is there. Whether society sees that or not is up for debate, but my experience is that the people who model for me inevitably see it, and the extent to which this seemingly subtle dance of photographer and model impacts their personal vision of themselves is exceedingly moving to me. It is a way of making a positive impact on the individual, as well as combating how limited the current beauty dictate happens to be.[17]

Rocker turned fatshionista, Beth Ditto, not only refuses to hide her size but flaunts it as the former lead singer of the indie rock band, *Gossip*. She quickly became a professional fashion designer. She has recently launched a clothing line geared toward women of size and cites her experience as a fat woman consumer who could not find desirable clothing for her size. Now, she both creates stylish clothing for fat women and models that very clothing in *haute couture* fashion shows.[18]

Ultimately, the Fat Acceptance movement's use of Signification is changing what it means to be beautiful and acceptable in American culture. It is changing what it means to be fat in our society. If beauty and fashion are genre sets in American culture, the privileged subject positions with access to those genres are changing through the infiltration of Fat Activism. Like a marginalized person using the Discourse of a dominant class, people of size are entering into fashion, modeling, and other aesthetic arenas in ways that challenge previously normalized players in the world of fashion, from creators to models.

Of course, the issue of racial marginalization remains and is a complicated intersection in the Fat Acceptance movement. Black women, for example, worked hard to seek representation in an already marginal movement. The success of Gabriel Sidebey and other black women of size have perpetuated myths that minority cultures already fully accept fat bodies. This is one of the reasons Fat Acceptance was predominately white for so long. The other, more salient reason seems to come out of old fashion racial and cultural insularity; blacks and whites often have a hard time fighting the general segregation of the society to which they are born.

My observation that the marginal nature of this movement in the larger racist society determined the nature of racial acceptance in the movement, suggesting the movement's acquisition of mainstream status may have to precede racial diversity to some extent. This has happened, to a degree. Of course, Fat Acceptance may not be at the center of hegemonic aesthetics, but it is now close enough, and racial diversity is now easier to bring along with it. Signification within Signification, then, was necessary and possible within the movement.

E. K. Daufin, professor of mass communication and cinematic studies at Alabama State University, often speaks of the racial significance of the Fat Acceptance movement, even if Giddens is not on her radar. When asked to consider symbolism regarding race, she says that the intersectional nature of Fat Acceptance—the confluence of race, sex, and body size—is not represented enough in either the language or symbols of Fat Acceptance.[19] The idea that fat bodies are more acceptable in minority cultures—a different interpretive community where symbols may change meaning—is debunked by Daufin.[20] Thus, Black women, too, are in need of fat positive Signification.

What Symbolism does for the activists and allies, alike, is show in certain terms that the visual and audible aspects of life are as important as the mental and intellectual aspects when it comes to creating change in the world.

DOMINATION AND THE FAT ACCEPTANCE MOVEMENT

Domination, according to Giddens, manifests as institutional backing in ways that overlap with respected hegemonic institutions, for example, academia and professional and activists organizations. The burgeoning field of Fat Studies has slowly grown out of women's studies and is intersectional with critical race theories, as well. Institutions like the National Association for the Advancement of Fat Acceptance (NAAFA) and the Association for Size Diversity and Health (ASDAH) echo the language of civil rights organizations meant to ensure human rights to the traditionally marginalized. Fat Acceptance, then, has institutional backing to fulfill Giddens requirement of dominance for societal acceptance.

Domination ensures a physical or virtual space where a community can feel supported and validated. Such places did not exist until the creation of NAAFA in 1969. This organization, in its initial manifestation, served merely to provide fat women with a place to fulfill both social and romantic wants and needs—such was the hostility and marginalization they met in mainstream society. This organization invited mostly fat women in order to encourage support and camaraderie, but it also invited men of various sizes who admired fat women (typically dubbed "fat admirers" or "F.A.'s"). Those interested in socializing but were more open to lesbian life styles created the Fat Underground. This movement, a bit more militant and politically active than the erstwhile social club of NAAFA, worked to empower women of size as worthy, aesthetically pleasing, and strong. The Fat Liberation Manifesto, an iconic document in the Fat Acceptance Movement penned by Judy Freespirit and Aldebaran, reads thus:

1. WE believe that fat people are fully entitled to human respect and recognition.
2. WE are angry at mistreatment by commercial and sexist interests. These have exploited our bodies as objects of ridicule, thereby creating an immensely profitable market selling the false promise of avoidance of, or relief from, that ridicule.
3. WE see our struggle as allied with the struggles of other oppressed groups against classism, racism, sexism, ageism, financial exploitation, imperialism, and the like.
4. WE demand equal rights for fat people in all aspects of life, as promised in the Constitution of the United States. We demand equal access to goods and services in the public domain, and an end to discrimination against us in the areas of employment, education, public facilities and health services.
5. WE single out as our special enemies the so-called "reducing" industries. These include diet clubs, reducing salons, fat farms, diet doctors, diet books, diet foods and food supplements, surgical procedures, appetite suppressants, drugs and gadgetry such as wraps and "reducing machines."
6. WE demand that they take responsibility for their false claims, acknowledge that their products are harmful to the public health, and publish long-term studies proving any statistical efficacy of their products. We make this demand knowing that over 99 percent of all weight-loss programs, when evaluated over a five-year period, fail utterly, and also knowing the extreme proven harmfulness of frequent large changes in weight.
7. WE repudiate the mystified "science" which falsely claims that we are unfit. It has both caused and upheld discrimination against us, in collusion with the financial interests of insurance companies, the fashion and garment industries, reducing industries, the food and drug industries, and the medical and psychiatric establishment.
8. WE refuse to be subjugated to the interests of our enemies. We fully intend to reclaim power over our bodies and our lives. We commit ourselves to pursue these goals together.
9. FAT PEOPLE OF THE WORLD, UNITE! YOU HAVE NOTHING TO LOSE.[21]

Although put forth by a faction of activism that would dissolve only a few years later, this text is seen as a manifesto for all fat activists in the present day. NAAFA has since grown into an activist and advocacy organization with an annual national conference. Its comprehensive website provides information on its mission, vision, and current activities. In line with its mission—"To eliminate discrimination based on body size and provide fat people with the tools for self-empowerment through public education, advocacy, and support"—and its vision—"A society in which people of every size are accepted with dignity and equality in all aspects of life"—NAAFA's activities range from providing a sanctuary of sorts for people of size weakened by societal animosity to providing education and advocacy for fat people and their allies.[22] In all, NAAFA aims to advocate for the following categories: activism, adoption and child custody discrimination, dieting and the diet industry, education, employment discrimination, fat people and the media, general well-being, obesity research, size-related legislation, weight-loss drugs, and weight-loss surgery. As one can see, NAAFA has come a long way since its early days as a social club.

Closely related to NAAFA is the Association of Size Diversity and Health (ASDAH). Often partnering with NAAFA, ASDAH promotes the aforementioned "General Well-Being" and "Obesity Research" topics emphasized by the former. In fact, the nutritionist behind ASDAH's Health At Every Size® Ideology—Linda Bacon—has been a steady contributor to both organizations. Bacon's book, *Health At Every Size*, is most influential to ASDAH's raison d'etre. The HAES® approach is thoroughly described on the comprehensive ASDAH website:

> The Association for Size Diversity and Health (ASDAH) affirms a holistic definition of health, which cannot be characterized as simply the absence of physical or mental illness, limitation, or disease. Rather, health exists on a continuum that varies with time and circumstance for each individual. Health should be conceived as a resource or capacity available to all regardless of health condition or ability level, and not as an outcome or objective of living. Pursuing health is neither a moral imperative nor an individual obligation, and health status should never be used to judge, oppress, or determine the value of an individual.
>
> The framing for a Health At Every Size (HAES®) approach comes out of discussions among healthcare workers, consumers, and activists who reject both the use of weight, size, or BMI as proxies for health, and the myth that weight is a choice. The HAES® model is an approach to both policy and individual decision-making. It addresses broad forces that support health, such as safe and affordable access. It also helps people find sustainable practices that support individual and community well-being. The HAES® approach honors the healing power of social connections, evolves in response to the experiences and needs of a diverse community, and grounds itself in a social justice framework.[23]

Linda Bacon, professor of nutrition and author of *Health At Every Size: The Surprising Truth about Your Weight*, explains that the reputation of fat as inherently unhealthy and fat people as unhealthy and ignoble is fed mostly by public assumptions that have been falsely presented as medical fact. Bacon writes that "much of what we believe to be true about weight . . . is in fact myth, fueled by the power of money and cultural bias."[24] Based on her government-funded, scientifically sound research on correlations of fat with health, she concludes thusly:

> Public health officials, health advocates, and scientists are complicit (often unintentionally) in supporting and encouraging the lies. The campaign against obesity is not about science or health; its misconceptions about the most basic research are astounding. If you suspend your preconceptions and open yourself to the scientific evidence, a very different picture emerges.[25]

Facts about health and weight are wildly overshadowed by the myths and lies about which Bacon and many others lament. Likewise, Paul Campos calls the ideal of obesity a faux disease[26] and that the correlations of "obesity" to health issues is too ambiguous to warrant legitimate medical diagnosis.[27] According to Campos and Bacon, the science behind the obesity epidemic is not just flawed; it may not even be science at all, since it seems to miss or ignore contradictory variables. The fact that ASDAH subsequently provides a list of HAES®-based healthcare workers strongly suggests that this mode of dominance—institutional backing—is working to break into mainstream discussions of health and fitness.

For a clue into how insidious and dangerous anti-fat sentiment can be in the healthcare field, one can look at *Love's Executioner,* a book of essays by writer and psychiatrist Irvin D. Yalom. When I came across the chapter titled "Fat Lady," I was initially delighted; I assumed this essay would be an exposition for psychiatrists and their fat patients about the psychological effects of being fat in a fat-hating society. Perhaps Yalom would draw attention to ways psychoanalysts inadvertently do more harm than good, offering, through intriguing narrative, ways to elude such situations. I assumed incorrectly. Yalom writes,

> I have always been repelled by fat women. I find them disgusting: their absurd sidewise waddle, their absence of body contour—breasts, laps, buttocks, shoulders, jawlines, cheekbones, *everything*, everything I like see in a woman, obscured in an avalanche of flesh. And I hate their clothes—the shapeless, baggy dresses or, worse, the tiff elephantine blue jeans with the barrel things. How dare they impose that body on the rest of us?[28]

Although he speaks in the present tense, I hoped this paragraph, found on top of the essay's second page, was an attempt at describing the mental and emotional obstacles Yalom would overcome to see the light of Fat Acceptance and, thus, become a better therapist. Again, I assumed incorrectly. Yalom's essay is about overcoming a mental block—the block of staying professional despite a severe disgust for one's client. The moral of this story is not that fat hate is bad, but that one can learn to work with a fat patient *despite* one's hatred for her. That is, a justified fat hatred should not trump one's professionalism. That is the point of the essay.

Yalom's client, named Betty, is guided by Yalom from the stereotypically jolly fat lady to a crazed dieter taking her anger toward society out on her body or, more specifically, her fat. The essay ends with a "touching" moment in which Yalom confesses his fat hatred and how it may have stifled his openness as a psychoanalyst. Betty responds in a calm and apparently undisturbed way. She soon explains her relatively unruffled demeanor in the following exchange with Yalom:

> "Remember when you were pushing me to go to Overeaters Anonymous? To meet other obese people—make some friends, get some dates?"
> "Yeah, I remember. You said you hated groups."
> "Well, that's true. I do hate groups. But it wasn't the whole truth. The *real* reason is that *I* can't stand fat people. They turn my stomach. I don't want to be seen with them. So how can I get down on you for feeling the same way?"[29]

The chapter ends with a good-bye hug that squeezes in one last bit of fat-bashing. Yalom writes, "When we embraced, I was surprised to find that I could get my arms all around her."[30]

What are we to make of this? Yalom's triumph is that he got past his client's disgusting body in an attempt to truly help her. The thought of getting past fat stigma, itself, was not an option.

Can we say that Yalom, like so many other people in health care, is as flawed as others conditioned to hate fat bodies? Yes. Can we say that Yalom's narrative is well-intentioned but tainted by societal misconceptions? Perhaps, but Yalom is a person responsible for assisting others in acquiring mental and emotional well-being. I am glad he was honest with himself and others about his feelings, but his fat hatred was not considered his flaw—the difficulty in ignoring his fat hatred was seen as the true weakness. Perhaps a civil but stern message to Yalom is in order.

I do not know Irvin Yalom. He seems to be a very accomplished man who has overcome much to acquire his success.[31] However, his ethos in his field and in his literary success makes his opinions about fat bodies all the more dangerous. Fortunately, more and more people are entering health care with HAES®-friendly and fat-friendly attitudes. The more vocal they are, the easier it will be to counter, if not reeducate, people like Yalom.

Yalom's professional expertise could not deter him from his learned fat hatred. Society allows such prejudice because anti-fat bias is seen, conversely, as pro-health support. Fat is directly correlated to, and seen as proof of, an unhealthy lifestyle, if not a lazy, ignorant, and immoral lifestyle. Thus, anti-fat bias, even at its worst, is often seen as a form of "tough love": the shaming of fat people into adopting a healthy lifestyle for their own good. Yet, this idea of tough love should be substantially deflated when anti-fat rhetoric comes up against ideologies like HAES®, which postulate that the popular correlations between weight and health are inconclusive, at best. If movements are considered anti-fat for the sake of fat people's health but dismissive of research that questions or disproves the automatic connection of a fat body to ill health, then that movement is less about health (and truth) and more about societal bias and, likely, monetary gain for the healthcare and weight-loss industries. In fact, insisting that a fat person is categorically unhealthy, lazy, immoral, or all of the above, when such a person, upon actual social and medical diagnosis, may be quite the opposite, can be construed as a form of slander, a mode of defamation, and an impingement on one's personal right to live one's own life. Although fat and health are considered antonyms in popular opinion, the inconclusive evidence regarding the correlations of fat to ill health renders anti-fat campaigns inherently defamatory.

An implied necessity of pragmatic change and Dominance as a helpful agent of change is the effective countering of opposing doctrines and ideologies. For an association like ASDAH, that would be the diet industry, in general. Battling a 60 billion dollar per year industry is difficult enough on its own. Battling such an industry and its federal backing, then, is quite the challenge. Beyond anti-fat sentiment from the former surgeon general who famously said that fat was the biggest national threat to America.[32] First Lady Michelle Obama's "Let's Move" campaign tends to perpetuate the idea that pro-health is primarily an avoidance of fat. "Let's Move" seems to present itself with rhetoric that seems to promote general health but, upon closer analysis, has weight loss as a primary focus. Michelle Obama's "Let's Move" campaign is a prime example of this. The home page for the Let's Move website seems to promote a healthy lifestyle, in general.[33] Links labeled "Eat Healthy" and "Get Active" seem to fall in line with the HAES® charge that health habits are the real goals and losing weight is not a panacea of fitness. Thus, the site seems to promote general health for all, making no claims that fat, per se, is the problem. However, upon clicking the "About Let's Move" link, one clearly can see that fat is construed as equal to, and directly the cause of, ill health. A link to the Childhood Obesity Task Force Report is placed above the following quote from First Lady Obama: "In the end, as First Lady, this isn't just a policy issue for me. This is a passion. This is my mission. I am determined to work with folks across this country to change the way a generation of kids thinks about food and nutrition."[34] As is explained in work by Bacon, Campus, Lyons and many others, one can adopt a lifestyle full of healthy choices about food and nutrition without losing weight or being considered "thin," but if the "Let's Move" campaign, backed by the highest office in the land, does not acknowledge that, fat activists have a long and arduous task ahead of them.

Upon clicking on the website's "Learn the Facts" link, a link typically meant to expound on the general ideology and mission of an organization, anti-fat initiatives abound, as well as several other links to articles specifically about childhood obesity. In fact, the prose in the "Learn the Facts" link is prefaced by another quote from the First Lady: "The physical and emotional health of an entire generation and the economic health and security of our nation is at stake."[35] Such a strong statement based on inconclusive evidence presented as hard fact is nothing fat activists aren't used to. The fact that it comes from the Oval Office, on the other hand, is especially daunting. The Strong4Life campaign, with its blatant move to agitate, is one thing. However, "Let's Move," backed by a beloved First Lady and wrapped in a rhetoric of progress, triumph, and heroism is much more difficult to combat.

So ASDAH must be as comprehensive and official as possible. The challenge, in fact, seems to have created the need and manifestation of a thorough organization that effectively combats the idea that a fat body is the unhealthy body of a lazy and undisciplined person. ASDAH's fact sheet, complete with scientific research backing the authenticity of the HAES® approach, is easily available. Resources in the following categories are also easily accessible: "Activism"; "Body Image"; "Children/Teens"; "Diabetes"; "Eating Disorders"; "Education"; "Exercise/Fitness"; "HAES® Science"; "Health Philosophy and Ethics"; "Health Policy, Law, and Legislation"; "Intersectionality"; "Mental Health/Psychology"; "Nutrition/Diet Related"; "Public Health and Health Promotion"; "Social Justice"; "Spirituality and Health"; "Stigma and Bias"; "Weight-Loss Surgery"; "Weight Science"; and "Workplace Wellness." These resources range from information documents to academic publications in the aforementioned fields. Thus, the effective overlap of institutions, that of civil rights, healthcare, and academia becomes more apparent.

Of course, an extension of ASDAH and its mission is the fair and equitable treatment of fat patients in the medical industry. Several stories exist of fat patients who went misdiagnosed for serious diseases because their physicians could not see past their size; "lose weight" would be the first and only prescription. What's more, dealing with fat, instead of looking for one's actual ailment, can lead to misdiagnosis and over-prescription of unnecessary medicines and procedures.[36] Scholars like Joan Chrisler and Angela Barney identify several instances in which this happens and see a dire need for a paradigm shift in the medical professions, citing the current trends in medicine, diagnosis based on body size, as inherently unethical and, surely, a form of malpractice.[37] Tracy L. Tylka et al. present the weight-inclusive/weight-normative to show the detriments of the former and the potential of the latter.[38]

Fortunately, health professionals who abide by the HAES®/Weight-inclusive paradigm do exist, thus opening the door to the aforementioned paradigm shift in institutions of medicine. In *Foundations for Community Health Workers*—a book that does not focus, specifically, on issues of size and health—Tim Berthold and Jill Tregor—provide health care professionals a bullet-pointed how-to for being properly weight-inclusive in their chapter titled "Promoting Healthy Eating and Active Living":

1. Do no harm
2. Appreciate that bodies naturally come in a variety of shapes and sizes, and ensure optimal health and well-being is supported for everyone, regardless of their weight.
3. Given that health is multidimensional, maintain a holistic focus.
4. Encourage a process focus (rather than end-goals) for day-to-day quality of life.
5. Critically evaluate the evidence for weight-loss treatment and incorporate sustainable, empirically supported practices in prevention and treatment efforts.
6. Create healthful, individualized practices and environments that are sustainable (e.g., regular pleasurable exercise, regular intake of foods high in nutrients, adequate sleep and rest, adequate hydration).
7. Where possible, work to increase health access, autonomy, and social justice for all individuals along the entire weight spectrum. Trust that people more toward greater health when given access to stigma-free healthcare and opportunities.[39]

Point 7 may be most salient for the criteria of Domination; it conveys a need to end inadvertent inequities concerning patient treatment.

Some health professionals not only abide by the HAES®/Weight-inclusive paradigm; they openly specialize in it. Besides Linda Bacon, Dr. DeAun Nelson of Watershed Wellness[40] and family nurse practitioner Shanti Herzog of Health Club, a fitness center in Portland, Oregon,[41] advertise themselves as body-positive healthcare professionals. Nelson's "focus is providing a safe place for people of all sizes to enjoy quality health care,"[42] while Herzog works at a center that focuses on giving "people of all shapes, sizes and identities the opportunity to learn transformative movement techniques with their friends in a fun and cozy environment."[43] Professionals like this are the trailblazers leading the medical professional into Fat Acceptance, which, in turn, will help provide Fat Acceptance with hegemonic Acceptance.

Kelly Bliss, therapist and exercise instructor who follows the HAES® model, has this to say about her methods when leading a workout:

> When doing a class, she speaks to everybody demographic. "Many people, when they come to my classes, have no idea I am a fat activist; they're actually shocked to see a fat instructor when they walk in, and they don't know that this class is anything about body Acceptance . . . all I do is talk neutrally about all types of body parts. If you have lean thighs, if you do [a] move be careful that you don't bump the bones of your knees together. If you have round and large thighs you have an advantage here because you can press against your softness and get extra resistance to develop your muscles. Those are true statements for any population, but they have inherent in them the Acceptance of all types of bodies.[44]

Fortunately, people like Kelly Bliss and others are becoming more numerous. Many also play dual roles as both healthcare professionals and academics. Linda Bacon, a professor at the City College of San Francisco, is just one healthcare professional who spends time in academia. In fact, the dual role of activist and scholar, in general, is becoming a norm within the movement. Thus, we come to another institution being infiltrated by the Fat Acceptance movement: academia.

Academia is the last strong institutional movement for Fat Acceptance, so far. The seeds of Fat Studies were initially planted by Susan Bordo and Susie Orbach. Bordo's *Unbearable Weight: Feminism, Western Culture, and the Body* addresses the stigma of fat and its effects on fat people, specifically fat women.[45] Orbach's *Fat is a Feminist Issue* directly uses the relative hegemony of feminist studies to draw attention to size discrimination and its origins in patriarchal dominance.[46] Although polemical, these books sparked a literary trend resulting in zines and anthologies of fiction and creative nonfiction. *Shadow on a Tightrope: Writings by Women on Fat Oppression*, is a 1983 anthology that worked to affectively begin the needed infiltration into academe. In the book's forward, Vivian Mayer writes that this book needs to be the first of many to solidify Fat Activism into an institution. After lamenting the rumors that Fat Acceptance groups all over the country started only to fold through in-fighting and the typical aggressions of isolation and anti-fat hostility. Mayer writes, "We will need more than the one anthology we now have. We will need more than a single book, or a single journal, or the support of a single feminist agency, none of which we have now. I pray for an outpouring of fat women's thought, speech, and action to come soon, in our days."[47] This, essentially, was a call to acquire Dominance.

This call seemed to initiate grassroots efforts to acquire Dominance. Zines like "Fat Girl" and "Size Queens" enjoyed a shifting level of popularity in Northern California as a place where people of size could express themselves and be heard by others.[48] These zines may have shared the literary realm of Fat Activism with more risqué magazines celebrating fat women as objects of beauty. Together, these works helped manifest Fat Acceptance as a genre in its own right. As with many popular forms of literature, its exploration and critique by academics was not far behind.

Books written by a variety of scholars both speak to Fat Studies' authenticity as a field and its necessarily interdisciplinary nature. Paul Campos, a lawyer, wrote *The Obesity Myth* to settle society misconceptions about the condition of fat bodies and lives.[49] Amy Farrell, an american studies/women's and gender studies scholar, wrote *Fat Shame: Stigma and the Fat Body in American Culture*, chronicling the initial stages of anti-fat sentiment in America from the nineteenth century to the present day.[50] Fat Studies scholars abound, and by this book's publication, more academics will have surely arrived.

Beyond literary anthologies that chronicle the fat experience, academic anthologies have become more abundant. *The Fat Studies Reader*, perhaps the most popular anthology to date, featured both activists and scholars of Fat Activism and Fat Acceptance.[51] The two-volume *The Politics of Size: Perspectives from the Fat Acceptance Movement*, meant to cater to a more eclectic audience of scholars and non-scholars, alike, followed just a few years later.[52] Shortly after its publication, the *Fat Pedagogy Reader*[53] was published, thus rounding out the academic significance of Fat Acceptance; it was a field with both theoretical and pedagogical presence in anthology form. That is, scholars were so steeped in the field that they were writing extensively on how to think about *and* teach Fat Studies.

Fat Studies is now a consistent area of study for the American Popular Culture Association's annual conference. The Fat Studies Conference, organized by Cat Pause of New Zealand's Massey University,[54] and the Fat Acceptance Conference organized by Ragen Chastain[55] are yearly and widely internet-streamed conferences that involve activists and scholars, alike. Consistent presence in a well-established national conference and standalone conferences on two continents speak to Fat Acceptance's embrace of Giddens's concept of Dominance.

Perhaps the most comprehensive take on Fat Studies comes from the rationale for the field, written by in the introduction to the first issue of *The Fat Studies Journal*. Editor, Esther D. Rothblum, writes, "Fat Studies scholars ask why do we oppress people who are fat and who benefits from the oppression. In that regard, Fat Studies is similar to academic disciplines that focus on race, ethnicity, gender, or age."[56] Thus, the precedent set by other "identity" studies, relatively hegemonic in status, gives Fat Studies the model and justification for its own existence. In fact, Fat Studies' aforementioned interdisciplinary nature may be the main conduit into academia. Interdisciplinarity gives Fat Studies its entry into several academic contexts, from a variety of disciplines to civic engagement. This desire to embrace several disciplinary Discourses and address the current academic concern of "impact" (the palpable influence of academia to society) gives Fat Activism a relatively smooth transition into academia.

Fat Studies is disciplinarily systemic within the liberal arts and impactful as an outgrowth of activism and advocacy for societal issues. The confluence of these outcomes—to be scholarly and impactful—matches well with a progressively common concept of the liberal arts. The 2008 Teagle Foundation white paper, "Liberal Education and the Preparation of Life and Work" created by the Teagle consortium consisting of several "liberal arts" institutions, identifies four concepts of liberal arts education to determine which ones would be most "impactful" to life and work preparation for students, which, of course, informs scholarly and administrative effectiveness. The consortium's description of liberal arts as a "mode of inquiry" describes many disciplines, but it's elaboration of this model bodes well for interdisciplinary fields. According to the Teagle Foundation,

> what is essential to this conception of liberal learning is the generalized intellectual lens that is brought to bear on an object of inquiry—one which places the subject matter in a socio-historical context; which pursues appropriate multiple cultural perspectives; which seeks to integrate multiple sources of knowledge, information, and expertise; and which cultivates an appropriate critical perspective.[57]

Fat Studies looks at the life experiences of fat from several lenses. From fiction to social sciences and hard sciences, the issue of fat is a fecund topic throughout academia. Giddens's Domination can be soundly justified.

LEGITIMATION AND THE FAT ACCEPTANCE MOVEMENT

Legitimation, for the purposes of Fat Acceptance, involves the legislation and policies necessary for the movement's success. That is, to be legal is to be legitimate. Laws ensuring equal rights for people of size have been fought for and won, thus pushing Fat Acceptance closer to hegemonic legitimacy. However, like many other forms of identity politics, a few victories are never enough. Fat activists work for legal rights in both the workplace and society.

Of course, winning in the law courts, per se, is not the real goal. Winning as an open and unashamed fat person is. As mentioned earlier, in "No Apology: Shared Stuggles in Fat and Transgender Law," Dylan Vade and Sondra Solovay compare two court cases in which both claimants were fat people suing for weight-based discrimination. One person, John, won over one million dollars, while the other, Toni, lost the case. Vade and Solovay seem to know the major difference between the cases.[58]

I return to Vade and Solovay to show that a lack of understanding at the legal level can have negative consequences for fat people who dare to think they have the rights to be listened to and treated like people. Although I am inclined to use the concept of defamation in this essay, I do not identify or seek to identify *legal precedents* involving defamation and size discrimination. In Toni's case, the employer's behavior is not a tort of defamation in the legal sense because an intentional misrepresentation of size/health correlations apparently was not proven. That is, the employer may have been mistaken, yet sincere. However, if proof that a fat body may not signal ill health or ignoble traits like hedonism, laziness, immorality, or ignorance is actively ignored by law courts as well as anti-fat campaigns, then a misrepresentation of facts and, therefore, a form of defamation—in its colloquial sense—may occur. In the framework of this chapter, a reference to Defamation law is best understood as a lens through which to see the nature and implications of anti-fat campaigns more clearly. So, if defamation in the strict legal sense is off the table, what are we talking about? One can conclude that Toni was defamed and that this defamation signals a need for policy changes that protect people of size.[59]

Like other marginalized groups, fat people are extremely underrepresented within the law. Ragen Chastain states "Discrimination due to weight is legal almost everywhere (exceptions being the state of Michigan and a handful of cities) I helped overturn a policy at Citizen's Medical Center to not hire healthcare professionals with a BMI over thirty-five because they believed that they failed to "fit with a representational image or specific mental projection for the job of a healthcare professional."[60] Ragen and fellow activists started an email campaign that pushed the Citizen's Medical Center to do away with the policy, thus showing the efficacy of Fat Activism's forays into Giddens's concept of Legitimation. That is, activism can legitimize people by altering laws and policies. This is imperative.

The ultimate key to success may be to educate legislators enough to have them pass laws that protect people of size regardless of their personal feelings about their weight. Of course, institutions and individuals exist who advocate for what is essentially fat civil rights. What's more, they have been successful. Nevertheless, more needs to be done.

We can easily identify current successes in policy. Laws do exist that protect fat people from weight-based discrimination. At the state level, only Michigan has anti-weight bias laws in place:

- Michigan is the only state with laws prohibiting discrimination against overweight people, which was enacted in 1977. The Elliott-Larsen Civil Rights Act prohibits discrimination practices based on ten categories, including weight.[61]

The following cities and towns have passed laws protecting fat people:

- Washington, DC: the Human Rights Law includes "personal appearance" in its protected categories.
- San Francisco, CA: the Human Rights Commission added "weight and height" to the municipal code to ensure that programs, services, and facilities would be accessible.
- Santa Cruz, CA: the municipal code on discrimination includes "height, weight, or physical characteristics" as protected categories.
- Binghamton, NY: the municipal code on discrimination includes "height, weight, or physical characteristics" as protected categories.
- Urbana, IL: the municipal code on discrimination includes "height, weight, or physical characteristics" as protected categories.
- Madison, WI: the municipal code on discrimination includes "height, weight, or physical characteristics" as protected categories.[62]

These are, indeed, victories. However, when compared to other equal rights legislation, fat activists have much more to accomplish.

Organizations dedicated to Fat Activism have been busy trying to secure protection by law. The National Association for the Advancement of Fat Acceptance (NAAFA) has an official stance on "Size-Related Legislation" that reads

> Because existing local, state, and federal statutes do not provide fat people with adequate protection from discrimination, NAAFA demands the inclusion of "height and weight" or "physical appearance" as a protected category and existing civil rights statutes and the enactment of additional laws as necessary to ensure protection against size discrimination in employment, education, housing, and public accommodations.[63]

What's more, NAAFA resolves to "actively support local, state, and federal anti-size discrimination legislation by providing background materials, writing letters of support, testifying, and/or engaging in public actions to the extent allowable by law."[64]

NAAFA recently published a document titled "Making a Case for Legislation to end Size Discrimination." NAAFA makes its case, perhaps most saliently, for fairness in the workplace and educational environments. Regarding the workplace, NAAFA provides the following statistics:

- Fat people can be terminated or suspended because of their weight, despite good job performance. (Rothblum, et al. 1990)
- Both men and women who were "obese" experienced lower wages compared to their "normal weight" counterparts. Fat women were paid 14.6 percent less than their "normal weight" counterparts. (Dor, et al. 2011)

- In the UK, 45 percent of 1,000 employers polled admitted they were less inclined to recruit at interview stage if the applicant was "obese." (Crossland Employment Solicitors Survey, 2015)
- Fat people get fewer promotions. (Loh, 1993)[65]

Regarding the primary and secondary school environment, NAAFA provides the following statistics:

- Negative attitudes start in preschool and progress as students age. (Turnbull, et al. 2000)
- 1 of 3 children has experienced weight bias from a teacher. (Rudd Report, 2008)
- In one study 28 percent of teachers said that becoming "obese" is the worst thing that can happen to a person. (Puhl and Brownell, 2001)
- In Elementary School, the likelihood of being bullied is 63 percent higher for an "obese" child than a "non-overweight" peer. (Lumeng, et al. 2010)
- Controlling for income and grades, parents provide less college support for their "overweight" children than for their "thin" children. (Puhl and Brownell, 2001)
- Higher BMI significantly predicted fewer post-interview offers of admission into psychology graduate programs. Results also suggest this relationship is stronger for female applicants.[66]

Although NAAFA encourages writing politicians to determine the correct stance on fat people's rights, the ASDAH has done so as an organization. This includes direct letters to presidential campaigns. The following excerpt is presented as a form letter to each candidate of the 2016 presidential election:

> Dear Candidate:
>
> I am writing for information on your stance with regard to adding "height and weight" or "size" to the anti-discrimination laws of this (city/state/nation). Discrimination based on body size has grown exponentially as anti-fat attitudes have taken root in our society. This issue is important to me personally and I would like to know if it is being included as a plank in your campaign platform.[67]

ASDAH has also published its letters to both the Senate and the House regarding the need for legislation against anti-fat tendencies in professional cultures. Generally, the letters warn against the misdiagnosis of medical patients based on weight, the use of a flawed diagnostic like BMI, and the dangers of workplace weight-loss programs that are often misinformed. Of course, the tenants of a HAES® approach to fitness is outlined and promoted. Other than a thorough review of the typical concerns of Fat Activism (unhealthy dieting, flawed diagnoses of health, etc.), the letter's salient point is conveyed below:

> We the leadership of the Association for Size Diversity and Health, an international organization composed of health professionals, scientists and activists committed to promoting all aspects of health and well-being for people of all sizes, are writing to express concern about weight-based language in the Senate Health Care Reform bill. We have serious concerns that weight loss will become institutionalized as a standard feature of prevention and wellness efforts. . . . Rather programs should encourage participation in healthy behaviors such as improved nutrition, increased exercise, stress reduction, and other activities known to promote health. We ask that any language in the final Health Care Reform bill limit programs, incentives and rewards to health-promoting programs rather than adherence to outcome criteria such as weight loss or BMI.[68]

Like much advocacy writing, such letters' very existence is a necessary step in the mainstreaming of social justice issues.

The most influential attempt at Legitimation and the mainstreaming of fat justice may come from another foray into the law courts. In the summer of 2016, *Playboy* model, Danie Mathers, photographed a picture of a fat woman showering in an LA Fitness locker room. She then put the picture on the internet with less than flattering things to say: "If I can't unsee this then you can't either."[69] Now she is facing a one million dollar lawsuit for violation of privacy. No, this is not a lawsuit against fat shaming, per se. However, the fact that an online petition to have Mathers brought up on charges, prompting the lawsuit, says much about the growing influence of fat activists and their sympathizers.[70] One signer of the petition, Heather Myers of Lakewood, California, has this to say:

> I'm signing this because Dani Mathers should be held responsible for this PREDATORY sex offense, just as any male who committed this same crime would be.
>
> I am signing this for all of the women out there who were already afraid to go to the gym because of something like this happening, who just had their worst nightmares confirmed.
>
> I am signing this to help make sure that NOTHING like this EVER happens again, and because Dani Mathers needs to be accountable for her disgusting and deplorable behavior.[71]

The effects of this incident could be a strong win for those against fat shaming and body shaming, in general. LA Fitness responded by issuing Mathers a lifetime ban from its facilities, saying, "Her behavior is appalling and puts every member's privacy at risk. We have handled this internally and also notified the police."[72] According to Jill Greuling, the company's executive vice president of operations, LA Fitness already has a policy banning cell phone use in the locker rooms, but her statement, "This is not only our rule, but common decency,"[73] may prompt other organizations to create clearer language on privacy, in general, and fat shaming, specifically.

No matter what happens with the Mathers case, fat people clearly are in need of legal protections in a variety of arenas. This third of Giddens's Structuration may be the most difficult, or at least the slowest, to accomplish substantially. Nevertheless, the steps are being taken to legitimize justice and equal rights for fat people.

NOTES

1. Marlow Stern. "Meet Ashley Graham, the *Sports Illustrated* Swimsuit Issue's First 'Plus-Size' Cover Girl," *The Daily Beast*, 17 Feb. 2016, accessed 28 Oct. 2016, http://www.thedailybeast.com/articles/2016/02/17/meet-ashley-graham-the-sports-illustrated-swimsuit-issue-s-first-plus-size-cover-girl.html.
2. Phil Wahba, "J.C. Penney Has Tapped This *Project Runway* Star to Launch Its Plus-Size Brand," *Fortune*, 12 Apr. 2016, accessed 27 Oct. 2016, http://fortune.com/2016/04/12/jc-penney-project-runway-ashley-nell-tipton/.
3. Margo Demello, *Body Studies: An Introduction* (New York: Routledge Press, 2014), 189–205.
4. Kelly Bliss, Interview, 31 July 2016.
5. Ragen Chastain, email message to author, July 28, 2016.
6. Ibid.
7. Jamar Nicholas, *BBWW: The Big Beautiful Wonder Woman Blog*, 20 Apr 2012, accessed 30 Oct. 2016, http://fatwonderwoman.blogspot.com/?view=classic.
8. Most famously, Wonder Woman graced the 1972 cover. The 40th anniversary of this cover is celebrated in an article from 2012: Kathy Spiller, "*Ms.* Turns 40 and Wonder Woman's Back on the Cover," *Ms Magazine Blog*, 1 Oct. 2012, accessed 28 Oct. 2016, http://msmagazine.com/blog/2012/10/01/ms-turns-40-and-wonder-womans-back-on-our-cover/.
9. Les Daniels, *Wonder Woman: The Golden Age*, (San Francisco: Chronicle Books, 2001), 26.
10. Deb Burgard, "The HAES® files: Stereotype Management Skills for HBO Viewers, *Health At Every Size® Blog*, 8 May 2012, accessed 28 Oct. 2016, https://healthateverysizeblog.org/2012/05/08/the-haes-files-stereotype-management-skills-for-hbo-viewers/.
11. *Weight of the Nation*, HBO, May 2012, accessed 30 Oct. 2016, http://theweightofthenation.hbo.com/.
12. Ragen Chastain, "Everybody Galileo Now," *Dances With Fat*, 7 May 2012, accessed 30 Oct. 2016, https://danceswithfat.wordpress.com/2012/05/07/everybody-galileo-now/.
13. Suzan Colon and Jennifer Traig, *What Would Wonder Woman Do?* (San Francisco: Chronicle Books, 2007), 53.
14. Substantia Jones, "The Adipositivity Project," Adipositivity.com, accessed 30 Oct. 2016, http://www.adipositivity.com/.
15. Substantia Jones, email message to author, 31 Aug. 2016.
16. "Noted Dicks at Tosh.0 Use Stolen Fat-Positive Photo to Make Fun of Fat People," *Jezebel.com*, 23 May 2012, accessed 30 Oct. 2016, http://jezebel.com/5912704/noted-dick-tosh0-uses-stolen-fat-positive-photo-to-make-fun-of-fat-people.
17. Velvet D'Amour, "Velvet," *Volup2*, 2015, accessed 30 Oct. 2016, http://www.volup2.com/velvet/.
18. Kristen Anderson, "Beth Ditto's Clothing Line Is Finally Here!" 12 Feb. 2016, accessed 30 Oct. 2016, http://www.vogue.com/13398654/beth-ditto-style-clothing-brand-plus-size-fashion/.

19. E. K. Daufin, Interview, 20 July 2016, accessed 2 Oct. 2016, https://www.dropbox.com/home?preview=Ek+Daufin.WAV.

20. Ibid.

21. Aldebaran and Judy Freespirit, "The Fat Liberation Manifesto," *The Fat Studies Reader*, ed. Esther Rothblum and Sondra Soladay (New York: New York University Press, 2009), 341–342.

22. NAAFA, "About Us," National Association for Advancement of Fat Acceptance, Inc., 2016, accessed, 31 Oct. 2016, http://www.naafaonline.com/dev2/about/index.html.

23. ASDAH, "HAES® Principles," Association for Size Diversity and Health, 2016, accessed 31 Oct. 2016, https://www.sizediversityandhealth.org/content.asp?id=76.

24. Linda Bacon, *Health At Every Size®: The Surprising Truth about Your Weight* (Dallas: Benbella Books, 2010), Kindle ed., ch. 6.

25. Ibid.

26. Paul Campos, *The Obesity Myth: Why America's Obsession with Weight Is Bad for Your Health* (New York: Gotham Books, 2004), 42.

27. Ibid.

28. Irvin D. Yalom, "Fat Lady," *Loves's Executioner* (New York: Basic Books, 2012), 94.

29. Ibid, 125

30. Ibid.

31. Irvin D. Yalom, "Curriculum Vitae," *Yalom.com,* accessed 1 Nov. 2016, http://www.yalom.com/pagemaker.php?nav=cv.

32. The Office of the Surgeon General, "The Surgeon General's Call to Action to Prevent and Decrease Overweight and Obesity," *National Center for Biotechnology Information*, 2001, accessed 31 Oct. 2016, https://www.ncbi.nlm.nih.gov/books/NBK44206/.

33. "Let's Move," *Letsmove.gov,* 2013, accessed, 31 Oct. 2016 www.letsmove.gov.

34. "About Let's Move," *Letsmove.gov,* 2013, accessed, 31 Oct. 2016, www.letsmove.gov/about.

35. "Learn the Facts," Let's Move! 2013, accessed 1 Nov. 2016, http://www.letsmove.gov/learn-facts/epidemic-childhood-obesity.

36. "HAES® Matters: Dieting, Disease, and Weight (Part 2)," *The Health At Every Size® Blog*, 23 Oct. 2012, accessed 1 Nov. 2016, https://healthateverysizeblog.org/2012/10/23/haes-matters-dieting-disease-and-weight-part-2/.

37. Joan Chrisler and Angela Barney, "Sizism Is a Health Hazard," in *The Fat Studies Journal: An Interdisciplinary Journal of Body Weight and Society*, 19 Aug. 2016, accessed 1 Nov. 2016, doi: 10.1080/21604851.2016.1213066.

38. Tracy L. Tylka et al., "The Weight-Inclusive versus Weight-Normative Approach to Health: Evaluating the Evidence for Prioritizing Well-Being over Weight Loss," *Journal of Obesity*, 2014, accessed 1 Nov. 2016, http://dx.doi.org/10.1155/2014/983495.

39. Tim Berthold and Jill Tregor, "Promoting Healthy Eating and Active Living," *Foundations for Community Health Workers*, 2nd edition, ed. Tim Berthold (San Francisco: Jossey Bass, 2016), 457–486.

40. ASDAH, "HAES® Expert DeAun Nelson," Association for Size Diversity and Health Inc., 2016, accessed 1 Nov. 2016, https://www.sizediversityandhealth.org/haes-expert.asp?id=202.

41. ASDAH, "HAES® Expert Shanti Herzog," Association for Size Diversity and Health Inc., 2016, accessed 1 Nov. 2016, https://www.sizediversityandhealth.org/haes-expert.asp?id=282.

42. ASDAH, "HAES® Expert DeAun Nelson."

43. ASDAH, "HAES® Expert Shanti Herzon."

44. Kelly Bliss, Interview, 31 July 2016.

45. Susan Bordo, *Unbearable Weight: Feminism, Western Culture, and the Body*, (Berkeley: University of California Press, 2003).

46. Susan Orbach, *Fat is a Feminist Issue* (London: Arrow Books, 2006).

47. Vivian Mayer, "Foreword," *Shadow on a Tightrope: Writings by Women on Fat Oppression*, ed. Lisa Schoenfielder and Barb Wieser (San Francisco: Aunt Lute Books, 1983), xvii.

48. Stefanie Snider, "Fat Girls and Size Queens: Alternative Publications and the Visualizing of Fat and Queer Eroto-politics in Contemporary American Culture," *The Fat Studies Reader*, ed. Esther Rothblum and Sondra Soladay (New York: New York University Press, 2009), 223–230.

49. Paul Campos, *The Obesity Myth: Why America's Obsession with Weight is Hazardous to Your Health*, (New York: Gotham Books, 2004).

50. Amy Farrell, Fat *Shame: Stigma and the Fat Body in American Culture*, (New York: New York University Press, 2011).

51. Esther Rothblum and Sondra Soladay, ed., *The Fat Studies Reader*, (New York: New York University Press, 2009).

52. Ragen Chastain, ed, *The Politics of Size: Perspectives from the Fat Acceptance*, (Santa Barbara, CA: Praeger Press, 2015).

53. *Fat Pedagogy Reader: Challenging Weight-Based Oppression through Critical Education,* (New York: Peter Lang Publishing, 2016).

54. Fat Studies Conference, Massey University, 2016, http://www.massey.ac.nz/massey/learning/departments/institute-of-education/events/fat-studies--identity-agency-and-embodiment/fat-studies--identity-agency-and-embodiment_home.cfm.

55. Fat Acceptance Conference, "Tools for the Revolution," https://fatactivismconference.com/.

56. Esther Rothblum, "Why a Journal of Fat Studies?" *The Fat Studies Journal*, ed. Esther Rothblum, 9 Feb. 2012, accessed 1 Nov. 2016, http://www.tandfonline.com/loi/ufts20?open=2.

57. Teagle Consortium. "Liberal Education and Preparation for Life and Work: A Teagle Foundation White Paper," *Teagle Foundation*, 5 Sept. 2008, accessed 1 Nov. 2016.

58. Dylan Vade and Sondra Solovay. "No Apology: Shared Stuggles in Fat and Transgender Law," in *The Fat Studies Reader* ed. by Esther Rothblum (New York: New York University Press, 2009), 168.

59. Emily Doskow, "Defamation Law Made Easy," *NOLO: Law for All*, 2005, http://www.nolo.com/legal-encyclopedia/defamation-law-made-simple-29718.html.

60. Ragen Chastain, email to the author, 1 Aug. 2016.

61. NAAFA, "Weight Discrimination Laws," National Association of Size Diversity and Health, Inc., 2016 accessed 31 Oct. 2016. http://www.naafaonline.com/dev2/education/laws.html.

62. Ibid.

63. NAAFA, "Size-Related Legislation," National Association of Size Diversity and Health, Inc., accessed 31 Oct. 2016. http://www.naafaonline.com/dev2/about/Policies/Size-Related_Legislation[2015].pdf.

64. Ibid.

65. NAAFA, "Making the Case for Legislation to End Size Discrimination," National Association of Size Diversity and Health, Inc., 2016 accessed 31 Oct. 2016, http://www.naafaonline.com/dev2/about/Brochures/NAAFA_Case_for_Legislation_2016.pdf

66. Ibid.

67. NAAFA, "NAAFA Newsletter," National Association of Size Diversity and Health, Inc., Sep. 2016 accessed 31 Oct. 2016, http://www.naafaonline.com/newsletterstuff/oldnewsletterstuff/September%202016%20NAAFA%20Newsletter.html#LETTER.BLOCK6)ASDAH.

68. ASDAH, "ASDAH Letter to the House," Association for Size Diversity and Health, 9 Feb. 2010, accessed 31 Oct. 2016, https://www.sizediversityandhealth.org/content.asp?id=205&articleID=71.

69. Madelyn Chung, "Playboy Model Dani Mathers Slammed for Publicly Body Shaming Nude Woman at Gym," *Huffington Post*, 15 July 2016, accessed 31 Oct. 2016, http://www.huffingtonpost.ca/2016/07/15/dani-mathers-body-shaming_n_11015320.html.

70. Jessica Perez, "Dani Mathers Should Be Arrested for Policy Violations," *Change.org*, 2016, accessed, 31 Oct. 2016, https://www.change.org/p/l-a-county-police-dani-mathers-should-be-arrested-for-privacy-violation.

71. Ibid.

72. Jessica Chasmar, " Playboy Playmate fired, banned for life from LA Fitness over locker room photo of naked woman," *Washington Post*, 15 July 2016, accessed 31 Oct. 2016, http://www.washingtontimes.com/news/2016/jul/15/dani-mathers-fired-banned-for-life-from-la-fitness/.

73. Veronica Rocha, "L.A. gym bans Playboy model after she posts body-shaming shower photo on Snapchat," *Los Angeles Times*, 15 July 2016, accessed 31 Oct. 2016, http://www.latimes.com/local/lanow/la-me-dani-mathers-body-shaming-gym-ban-20160715-snap-story.html.

Chapter Three

Fat Tactics and the Pragmatics of Fat Activism

As one can discern, Structuration is an end, but the means to that end is pragmatic activism. What we see in Giddens's Structuration can help us better understand the successes of Fat Activism. We see how Signification, Dominance, and Legitimation have been vehicles to help people of size enter into hegemony. However, the application of Structuration to Fat Activism does not tell the whole story. Fat Activism, as an activist movement, had to utilize—advertently or inadvertently—certain strategies to acquire the presence and ethos it currently enjoys. To get closer to this hegemony and make it more inclusive, these tactics need to be perpetuated relentlessly. That is, agitation, described as a prolonged resistance using unorthodox rhetorical strategies, needs to be maintained. But, in addition, the movement needs to appreciate a level of pragmatism as well. Agitation without pragmatism could be construed as grandstanding, self-adulation, or—at worst—the tantrums of an unpopular minority.

In order to see where Fat Activism has gone and can go from here, an exploration of activism, itself, may be in order. This chapter, and much of the book's remainder, will argue the imperative role of pragmatism in current modes of Fat Activism. At the risk of seeming prescriptive, I will show how a sustained activism has to be a future of applied pragmatism and perlocutionary or instrumental activism[1] in addition to esteem building and consciousness raising activities. By no means am I saying that Fat Acceptance does not do this already; its current successes are a result of applied pragmatism. I am merely describing what has happened and what needs to continue happening to stave off entropy and perpetuate success.

As a framework on understanding the kinds of activism that help accomplish Giddens's Structuration, I look to the work of activist Jonathan Smucker. His experience as an activist has led him to write *Hegemony How-To: A Roadmap for Radicals* and create "Beyond the Choir," an organization that helps educate and train people in the creation and successful execution of social movements. I use Smucker's work because it aligns nicely with what has worked in Fat Activism but may also suggest ways the movement could improve by eliminating aspects that could be construed as obstacles.

Smucker, who uses the successes and failures of activist endeavors, most saliently the Occupy Wall Street movement, as a cautionary tale for fighting against subjectivity, insularity, and exorbitant identity politics to better ensure concrete results. Ultimately, one can glean the importance of pragmatic thinking, as opposed to self-righteous ideation, in advancing Fat Acceptance. This pragmatism may not sound ideal to many, especially those who mainly focus on the identity politics and esteem building aspects of Fat Activism. However, through an objective observation of activism, one can see the necessity of combining mental and emotional uplift with tactical pragmatism. Smucker provides the framework for successful activism. Fat activists, themselves, will fill that framework with works and actions that strengthen and perpetuate the movement. Through such pragmatic activism, we can arrive at Structuration more effectively.

Let us look at activism as an esteem movement. Some players in Fat Acceptance, who I will call "esteem-activists" abide by modes of activism meant to awaken fat people, especially fat women, to the idea that they have been duped into abiding by an arbitrary hegemonic aesthetic. As discussed when outlining the place of Giddens's concept of Signification and Dominance in Fat Acceptance, we see symbols that help fat people, themselves, rise into self-acceptance. Much, if not most, of the Fat Acceptance movement is based on the goal of esteem building, and for good reason. If people want to push a society to accept currently marginalized people, those people would do well to convince those very marginalized people that they, themselves, are worthy of the respect afforded to more hegemonic players. Fat Acceptance cannot thrive without fat people who have already accepted themselves. Thus, the movement needs to expose hegemonic aesthetics as an arbitrary part of an American (at least) metanarrative that demonizes fat in several ways (aesthetically, morally, intellectually, etc.). Based on this metanarrative, to be fat is to be un-American. It is to lack virtue or the right to be a respected citizen. Demystifying this overarching ideology to those most detrimentally affected by it—fat people and, to an extent, those who love fat people to any capacity—is imperative to taking the first steps in the Fat Acceptance movement.

Of course, esteem activism is a necessary end in itself, but it must not be an end in the grand scheme of Fat Acceptance in America. Depending on context, esteem activism may be less of an end and more of a means. Smucker distinguishes between an end goal and a tactic—a step toward an end goal—in his work: “A tactic is basically an action taken with the intention of achieving a particular goal, or at least moving toward it. . . . A successful tactic is one that sets us up to eventually achieve gains that we are not presently positioned to win.”[2] Although esteem activism is an important and necessary step in Fat Activism, it can double as a tactic toward a more profound telos that secures all aspects of Structuration.

Smucker suggests that many activist movements fail because activists stop at esteem politics for its own sake. For those activists, the symbolism of an event, a piece of art, or a written text is enough. The very existence of those things are victories in themselves. According to Smucker, these things must be prepared to hold dual positions as both ends and means in a bigger teleological struggle.

We have already looked at some actions within the Fat Acceptance movement that have been very powerful as esteem builders, securing both pride and agency to people of size. We discussed Substantia Jones’s Adipositivity, and the Big, Beautiful Wonder Woman phenomenon, but several other movements exist to help fat people combat hegemonic oppression. The “Fuck Yeah” blog series and “Fat People Flipping You Off” are two websites dedicated to showing images of fat people defiantly flouting anti-fat sentiments. They are popular and almost self-perpetuating actions within Fat Acceptance.

The “Fuck Yeah” series of fat activist blogs is quite popular. From “Fuck Yeah, Fat Postivity” to “Fuck Yeah, Fat Cosplay,” the websites celebrate the simple idea of fat people enjoying their lives, hobbies, and occupations (“Fuck Yeah, Fat PhDs” also exists) without concern for their body size or the negative characteristics projected onto them by society. They may be interpellated in negative ways by an anti-fat ideology, but they seem to create their own narrative and happily live within that world where fat is not just normal but a cause for celebration.

Most “Fuck Yeah” sites do not provide much in the way of a mission statement; perhaps the images and comments speak for themselves. However, “Fuck Yeah, Fat Haircuts” does provide a short but powerful narrative that attracts frustrated fat women via what John W. Bowers et al. would call “referent power”: a force that attracts powerless people with the implicit promise of providing strength to those in want of it.[3] The narrative starts with a sample of typical anti-fat—if passive-aggressive—statements before getting to the crux of the site’s mission: “You have such a pretty face, but that haircut makes it look so round. I don’t think that cut is right for your . . . um, bone structure. I’m not sure you have the face for bangs. Seriously, fuck that. This is the place to see awesome hair styles on awesome fatties. ANY face can rock ANY hair . . . it’s just up to you.”[4] As you can see, the narrative ends with a rejection of an apparently recognizable story, serving as a kind of metonym for society’s policing of fat bodies. This site is clearly a place to find like-minded people—people made to feel ashamed of their bodies—created by people who are frustrated about having to feel ashamed of their bodies. This site is a sanctuary, a space borne of esteem activism.

According to the creators of "Fat People Flipping You Off," the site's purpose is a simple but necessary rhetoric of defiance:

> What is FatPeopleFlippingYouOff.com? It's fat people. Flipping you off.
>
> Fat people who're angry about sizeism, both institutional and individual. Cheesed off about revisionist science, body policing, and implicit weight bias. Pissed about the $66 billion/year US weight loss industry blanketing media with dangerous messages meant to convince people they're inadequate and unworthy simply because their bodies occupy the larger end of natural human variation.[5]

This website represents a collective scream of "We're not gonna take it!" The empowerment is evident in the photos. The sense of belonging is evident in the sheer number of photos (the archives seem to go back two years, but the site may be older than that).

The "Fuck Yeah" and "Fat People Flipping You Off" sites can be seen in two ways. First, each can be seen as an end in promoting esteem and a sense of belonging to something that could replace feelings of helplessness with feelings of power, that is, "referent power." According to Smucker, movements stagnate because many people find a sense of belonging and are so satiated that they do not think of moving on. They may even bristle at the idea of progressing tactically based on a need to make the best of a newly acquired comfort zone to build necessary alliances.[6] I have met people who do enjoy Fat Acceptance but do not wish to go any further than the personal acceptance of their own bodies. Others want to focus on rescuing fat people from social stigma and raise consciousness about the arbitrary nature of hegemonic aesthetics. These things are fine and necessary. To Smucker, this activism is akin to therapy; this is good a thing.

Yet, the sites can also be seen as tactics to agitate those who harbor anti-fat sentiments and get a conversation going about the motivations and goals of those who would create such websites. Ways to build on the sites depend on the particular rhetorical situation; one must gauge a particular audience and understand its relationship to a subject or a symbol of a subject before effectively addressing it. However, the point is that the sites move from therapeutic to tactical, from collective ritual to strategic engagement.[7]

I am not sure if the sites' administrators or most of the sites' members see the sites as both therapeutic and tactical, but the potential is there. Recognizing this potential is imperative to successful activism. The administrators of "Fat People Flipping You Off" do discuss talking points in their "About" page and provide a well-known—though uncited on the site—statistic about the weight-loss industry's profits, thus pointing their middle fingers at neoliberalism at large. But the monological nature of an "About" page could become tactical if used as a prompt for dialogue.

An example of esteem activism becoming strategic engagement can be seen through an incident involving the "Fuck Yeah, Fat PhDs" site. In 2013, Geoffrey Miller, a psychology professor at the University of New Mexico, tweeted "Dear obese PhD applicants: if you didn't have the willpower to stop eating carbs, you won't have the willpower to do a dissertation #truth."[8] The tweet received immediate attention from several publications—including the *Huffington Post*, the *Atlantic*, *Inside Higher Ed*, and the *New Yorker*—and actually prompted the creation of "Fuck Yeah, Fat PhDs" several days later. One could see this as an example of esteem activism only, but that would be a neglect of the big picture. Several "Fuck Yeah" sites had already been up. Miller's tweet, which garnered critical responses from people inside and outside the Fat Acceptance community, may have been the catalyst for "Fuck yeah, Fat PhDs"[9] but the seed of activism—the motivation to not just feel good but fight back—was already there and put there by sites like "Fuck Yeah" and "Fat People Flipping You Off." Cat Pausé, a professor at New Zealand's Massey University who organizes an annual conference of Fat Studies, created "Fuck Yeah, Fat PhDs." Her rationale speaks to Miller's role in this activist space.

> This is not about this one guy who tweeted this one hateful thing—it's about our larger culture and how we are content to allow fat individuals to exist as second class citizens. Buy a second plane ticket, pay more for healthcare, only be represented in the media in a negative fashion—all of these are regular parts of life for fat people and very few seem to care.
>
> I'm not interested in responding to Dr. Miller. While I appreciate those who want to call him out, and yes he deserves it, I'm more interested in addressing the social narratives in which individual comments like Dr. Miller's are encouraged. I'm also interested in the structural aspects of fat oppression. I decided that what I wanted to do was to highlight all the amazing fat individuals who are in graduate school, or have completed graduate school—to provide a visual repository for anyone who doubts that fat individuals lack the abilities or qualities to succeed in academia. And to celebrate the amazing work being done by these rad fatties![10]

So, the incident prompted esteem activism while also creating an opportunity—granted, one buttressed by national media attention—to make more people aware of the negative and inequitable effects of fat discrimination. Smucker would see this as ideal activism: one incident doubling as therapeutic and tactical depending on the rhetorical situation, ready to float from one role to the other.

THE PRAGMATICS OF ALIGNMENT

A large part of the success of "Fuck Yeah, Fat PhDs" comes from the fact that the incident was covered by various popular news outlets. In a sense, fat activists used this as a vehicle to get more information to the masses about the very existence of Fat Acceptance. Geoffrey Miller's tweet was a catalyst that sparked an activist surge that was already progressing; it was the rain to a seed that had already breached the surface of the soil. However, if fat activists were to wait for celebrity insults to take advantage of national exposure, the movement may not move as far or as quickly as it could. This is why the concept of alignment is a key to successful activism.

According to Smucker, political alignment is a consummate example of pragmatic activism: an act of joining forces with previously established institutions that share enough values and goals to create a new, stronger "we." The larger the *viscera pisces* in the Venn Diagram of two separate institutions, the stronger the alignment. Giddens's concepts of Domination and, as I will show, Legitimation often rely on this kind of alignment. Smucker's definition of political alignment is worth quoting.

> An alignment of different social groups, organizations, and movements into a unified force that intervenes to shape social, economic, and political reality. I use this term to describe both the process of aligning otherwise fragmented groups, and also the force or vehicle that, once aligned, can contend in the *hegemonic contest*. Such an alignment is not necessarily clearly defined, neatly delineated, or formally coordinated; often it is none of these things. A political alignment stays intact to the extent that its component parts identify with or see their interests bound up with it.[11]

Smucker defines two kinds of alignment, *challenger alignment* and *hegemonic alignment*, meant to alter the status quo or make the status quo more inclusive, respectively.

This concept of political alignment is why I cite the Fat Acceptance movement in conjunction with movements like the Body Positivity movement and the HAES® movement. Fat Acceptance activists often dismiss these movements because aspects of their core ideologies often obscure goals of Fat Acceptance. Body Positivity's focus on all bodies takes necessary energy away from the bodies most maligned in our society: fat bodies. In addition, HAES® may suggest that being fat is only okay if you actively exercise and eat a certain way, implying that fat people who don't do so deserve less respect. Although these disparities, actual or perceived, are important and should not be ignored, political alignment asks activists to gauge sites of activism and discern how a partnership of these movements may be utilized in a tactical way. That is, for pragmatic purposes contingent of the situation, utilize the *viscera pisces* that will advance activists goals. Alignment is key to acquiring Giddens's Domination and Legitimation. Differences should not be ignored, but similarities should be utilized as strategically as possible.

An example of political alignment in Fat Activism can be seen with the effective partnership of the Fat Acceptance movement with the Americans with Disabilities Act. This partnership did not come about without some controversy. At the very least, calling fat a disability was received as an insult by both fat activists (especially those based firmly in esteem building) and people deemed disabled in a more traditional sense (especially those who deem fatness a "choice" rather than a "condition"). However, choosing the proper frame through which to view fatness and disability simultaneously was a key tactic to accomplishing Giddens's Legitimation.

First, significant differences exist between bodies designated "fat" and those designated "disabled" from a societal (and stereotypical) standpoint. A major difference between society's view of disabled bodies and fat bodies is the conception that fat people are "to blame" for fat, suggesting character flaws, not unfortunate circumstances, cause fat bodies. Pattie Thomas, in *Taking Up Space: How Eating Well and Exercising Regularly Changed My Life*, writes that being fat is a potentially silencing effect, because, to many people (including those deemed disabled) a fat body is considered proof of incompetence, laziness, and so forth.[12] Where disabled people are considered heroes or martyrs for daring to live their lives (not an unproblematic sentiment, itself), fat people are considered in completely opposite terms.

This being said, many fat activists and scholars acknowledge some parallels between the stigmatization suffered by fat people and that suffered by the disabled. To clarify, bodies deemed "disabled" by the Americans with Disabilities Act, have to abide by at least one of the following criteria: (A) "a physical or mental impairment that substantially limits one or more of the major life activities of such individual"; (B) "a record of such an impairment"; or (C) "being regarded as having such an impairment."[13] Based on this definition, newly constructed in 2008, extremely tall people could be considered disabled *in certain contexts*. So, one can see how the ADA can overlap Fat Acceptance and how Disability Studies could inform Fat Studies. Like the term "disabled," "fat" is seen as a condition that impedes physical activities that it actually does not. For one, many fat people are "able-bodied" in that often they out-perform their thinner counterparts.

As you can see, the alignment of Fat Activism and the Americans with Disabilities Act had potential to crash and burn; redefining fat as a "disability" could have weakened the necessary esteem movements that had gotten Fat Activism so far. However, working from the terministic screen of "societal" disability instead of "individual" disability not only maintained pride and esteem within the movement, but helped the movement acquire legal, political, and occupational protection. This is alignment at its best.

Fat Studies scholar Charlotte Cooper discusses the efficacy of the alignment between the ADA and the Fat Acceptance movement. In her *Disability and Society* journal, "Can a Fat Woman Call Herself Disabled," Cooper explains her surprise when realizing that fat people and disabled people had significantly similar experiences based on the "social model of disability"[14] articulated as criteria "C" in a previous paragraph. She acknowledges, then, that identification (i.e., alignment) with the disabled is a political move based on real similarities and the precedential successes of disability politics.[15]

Framing disability, or at least a large segment of disability, as a "society" problem is key to the alignment of Fat Acceptance activism and Disability Studies. Yet, those who identity more with criteria A and B of the disability definition may see this alignment as more of an appropriation. Cooper addresses this. She writes, "The notion of jumping on a bandwagon here implies that the social model is [disabled people's] work, something which belongs to 'them,' not 'us' and this further establishes the conceptualization of disabled people as 'other.' It also implies ownership and relevancy to one section of society, rather than a theory which is more universally applicable and useful."[16] Thus, the relegation of identity politics may be antithetical to all parties if it is in their best interest to change society to be more inclusive. In fact, Smucker cites exclusivity as a primary reason for a movement's failure.[17] Partnerships, or "challenge alignments" are ideal when the problem is an oppressive societal ideology. Put simply, there is power in numbers.

So, we can see why alignment is a powerful political move for both parties. For Fat Acceptance, the major impetus for identifying as disabled is to get a foot in the door of social consciousness. Fat Activism is considered laughable while Disability Studies, even if still misunderstood, is taken seriously as a legitimate and necessary endeavor. To join the Disability movement is to ensure a voice and visibility, even if a terministic screen of disability invites unwanted attention. Regarding the unwanted attention the disability movement may want to avoid by excluding fat people, the synthesis of people and resources may justify partnership. Using a sports metaphor, Smucker writes that "if a movement wants to score any goals, it needs to see and value *other groups* as players on the same team, moving the ball in the same general direction."[18]

Perceived differences from society and between fat and disability politics focus on the intellectual and moral characteristics attributed to people of size. On the other hand, people of size who were fighting for fat pride and the perpetuation of the idea that all bodies are normal and natural bodies may shy from the term disabled for its connotations of being "less than." Secondly, although fat people are ostracized, they are rarely segregated "for their own good" like disabled people. Thus, Cooper implores activists on both sides to not only work together, but "see" together. Cooper wants to change the frame on disability. If both parties critiqued the criticisms, they could both reconstruct disability in a way socially beneficial to both parties.[19]

Thus, Cooper shines light on the similarities between fat and disability politics. Most clearly, and, again, exposed by the social model of disability, both fat and disabled people share low status in society. Both experience a lack of access in society—from clothing to comfortable seating—thus feeling unwanted. Both parties are unfairly medicalized. We discussed the medicalization of fat even with proof that suggests fat does not objectively determine ill health. However, in disability politics, similar misdiagnosis takes place under the guise of sympathy; this is called "the personal tragedy" model of disability. This model "implies that the experience of disability is deeply traumatic and that the disabled individual must be rehabilitated to become a useful member of normal, able-bodied society."[20] This model does two things: it segregates disabled people who do not want or necessarily need to be segregated into institutions meant to specialize in their issues; and it creates a perception of disabled people that perpetuates a weakness, helplessness, and uselessness that is often quite inaccurate.

So, although fat people are often blamed for their conditions, both parties suffer an "invasive pity" ubiquitous in the Western world.[21] Both parties align because the social model puts them in shared space as people unnecessarily marginalized from society because of their bodies or perceived abilities. Thus, disability, like fatness, is the experience of social oppression and discrimination. Cooper, then, adopts a disabled identity because she feels impaired by societal oppression. This alignment, actually legitimated by the ADA, itself, via Criteria "C," has assisted in acquiring Giddens's Legitimation.

As powerful as alignment can be, obstacles do come into play. First, many within the Fat Acceptance movement were not happy with deeming fat bodies as "disabled." According to Anna Kirkland, professor of women's studies and political science, "If fat people were to gain ADA protections, then, this critical perspective would predict that they would exchange moral condemnation for the typical 'personal tragedy' story of people with disabilities, understood as unfortunate souls afflicted with a lamentable condition beyond their control. The focus would remain on their bodily or genetic impairments, because the danger is that most people still think of disabilities in that way."[22] This sentiment stems from many people's lack of awareness of the social model of disability, which posits society, not people, as the disabled entity. That is, because society is so restricted, a fat person's activities within it are hindered. This take on the definition of disability is key.

Kirkland, however, differs on this. She worries that the ADA's focus on employment stops there; its protections cannot be parlayed into social awareness and the creation of an identity group. She cites the concept of "individualized management," that is, the act of dealing with each individual case through an interactive process specific to that particular case, as antithetical to creating the unified group needed for most fat activist goals.[23] In this case, a case-by-case, social epistemic way of doing things is ideal for an individual worker—the point of ADA—but not for a movement trying to spread awareness about the societal misconceptions of fat people and fat bodies.

I am inclined to disagree with Kirkland from a pragmatic perspective. Alignment between disabled people and fat people are important, if only for workplace protections and accommodations. However, from a pragmatic and goal-oriented perspective, a social-epistemic approach may be ideal. James Berlin's description of social-epistemic rhetoric is worth quoting at length.

> Social-epistemic rhetoric is self-reflexive, acknowledging its own rhetoricity, its own discursive constitution and limitations. This means that it does not deny its inescapable ideological predispositions, its politically situated condition. It does not claim to be above ideology, a transcendent discourse that objectively adjudicates competing ideological claims. It knows that it is itself ideologically situated, itself an intervention in the political process, as are all rhetorics. Significantly, it contains within it a utopian moment, a conception of the good democratic society and the good life for all its members. At the same time, it is aware of its historical contingency, of its limitations and incompleteness, remaining open to change and revision.[24]

Combining a pragmatic attitude with social-epistemic rhetoric, then, is to never settle for any particular strategy beyond its immediate use. A strategy's or tactic's efficacy is kairotic, that is, contingent upon a rhetorical situation. Criteria "C" can support group identity if the situation is gauged right and Aristotle's understanding of rhetoric efficacy—discerning the "available means of persuasion"—are taken seriously. To put it simply, one need only wait for the prudent occasion to utilize Criteria "C" as a heuristic of sorts. The confluence of Fat Activism and the ADA will benefit fat employees, individually. However, as a precedent for supporting the importance of societal influence on ideologies of ableism, Criteria "C" will have its moments of relevance, its moments of strategic alignment. Thus, to put things in Smucker's terms, the ADA—the social model of disability, specifically—is not an end goal but a tactic, a step, toward the end goal: societal acceptance and respect.

The alignment of Fat Activism with the ADA is a challenger alignment; it is meant to change society into one that is more inclusive. This means challenging the terministic screen through which we, as a society, have been viewing fat. In essence, fat activists align with the ADA's social model of disability to say to hegemony, "It's not us; it's you." This sentiment is solidified in the ADA for those with disabilities. Alignment would open the door for Fat Acceptance.

All of this is to show that change depends on pragmatic strategy. Of course, identity politics and movements to enhance esteem are important for Fat Activism, but it is a first step toward creating concrete change, not the *telos* some activists deem it to be. To do this, movements would do well to be both therapeutic (esteem-building) and tactical. This is seen in "Fuck Yeah, Fat PhDs" which serves as both an esteem-building movement and a movement to promote societal awareness of Miller's ill-advised assessment of fat people in education. "Fuck Yeah, Fat PhDs," then, made the best of a kairotic moment—Miller's tweet and its backlash—to do important activist work.

Alignment, then, is a pragmatic strategy for activism. Although I focus on Fat Activism's alignment with the ADA, other modes of alignment—especially in academia—are also taking place. These alignments are not perfect—some people in both camps may be opposed to the partnerships for various reasons—but the strategy is pragmatically sound.

The internal problems in Fat Acceptance are just one of many obstacles to the movement, most of which are external to the movement. In the next chapter, I want to focus on the impetus and nature of these obstacles—road blocks on the way to accomplishing Giddens's Structuration—and what is being done to overcome them.

NOTES

1. Perlocutionary force is derived from J. L. Austin's work in sociolinguistics. A perlocution is a statement that results in an actual action. John W. Bowers et al. describe this phenomenon as an instrumental act and applied more directly to concrete results is activism, specifically.
2. Jonathan Matthew Smucker, *Hegemony How-To: A Roadmap for Radical* (Chica, CA: AK Press, 2017), 56.
3. John W. Bowers, Donavan J. Ochs, Richard J. Jensen, David P. Schulz, *The Rhetoric of Agitation and Control,* (Long Grove, IL: Waveland Press, 2010), 15.
4. *Fuck Yeah, Fat Haircuts,* http://fuckyeahfathaircuts.tumblr.com/.
5. "About," *Fat People Flipping You Off,* http://fatpeopleflippingyouoff.tumblr.com/about.
6. Smucker, 83–84.
7. Ibid., 79.
8. Laurent Ingeno, "Fat-Shaming in Academe," www.insidehighered.com. June 4, 2014.
9. Ibid.
10. Cat Pausé, "Fuck Yeah, Fat PhDs," *Friends of Marilyn*, June 30, 2015.
11. Smucker, 264.
12. Pattie Thomas, *Taking Up Space: How Eating Well and Exercising Regularly Changed My Life* (Nashville, TN: Pearlsong Press, 2013), LOC. 500, Kindle edition.
13. The United States Department of Justice-Civil Rights Division, AMERICANS WITH DISABILITIES ACT OF 1990, AS AMENDED, https://www.ada.gov/pubs/adastatute08.htm#12101.
14. Charlotte Cooper, "Can a Fat Woman Call Herself Disabled?, *Disability and* Society 12, No. 1, 1997, 32, DOI: 10.1080/09687599727443.
15. Ibid., 31.
16. Ibid., 33.
17. Smucker, 96.
18. Ibid., 97.
19. Cooper, 36.

20. Ibid.
21. Ibid., 38.
22. Anna Kirkland, "What's at Stake in Fatness as a Disability?" *Disability Studies,* 26, No. 1, 2006, http://dsq-sds.org/article/view/648/825 .
23. Ibid.
24. James Berlin, *Rhetoric, Poetics, and Culture* (TK), 81.

Chapter Four

Anti-fat Rhetoric and Social Media

Charges against the Fat Acceptance movement and the Health At Every Size® concept are well-known and well-chronicled within Fat Activism and Fat Studies. As discussed in the introduction to this text, an eclectic group of activists, scholars, health professionals, and lawyers discuss the misrepresentation of the cause and effect relationship between weight and health. Much time and energy has been spent on illuminating these misrepresentations as obstacles to Fat Acceptance. As I discussed in the previous chapter, workplace discrimination based on aesthetic preferences also presents itself as an obstacle that needs to be overcome. Social media representation, agitation, and alignment are some of the ways that activists have attempted to overcome these roadblocks to acceptance.

The internet has been a favored tool for many activists and fat activists are no exception. However, along with internet representation comes consequences. Like fat activists, anti-fat trolls also have access to the internet, especially its comment sections. Many troll groups, consisting of people both aware and unaware of concepts like Health At Every Size® and the Fat Acceptance literature, have popped up for the sole purpose of discouraging or ruining the efforts of fat people and fat activists to acquire group pride and societal success. My argument is that internet trolls are the frontline of anti-fat rhetoric and, thus, must be addressed as readily as health and workplace discrimination.

Trolls, or those who, according to Merriam-Webster, "attempt to antagonize (others) online by deliberately posting inflammatory, irrelevant or offensive comments or other disruptive content," are not necessarily a new phenomenon. In a sense, they are run-of-the-mill bullies in "cyber" form. From behind a keyboard—as opposed to face-to-face—trolls seek to create arguments for two major reasons: to hurt others and to maintain or fabricate a sense of power. So, the schoolyard bullies who consistently picked on the fat kids (or any kids outside of what the bullies deemed normal) are enjoying a more contemporary, global, and anonymous medium. Generally, I am interested in the concept of trolling because I think it provides insight into the ubiquitous cruelty of contemporary American culture, but also because the most vicious attacks on those trying to promote and exude fat pride, or even body positivity, come in the form of faceless internet harassment.

In fact, I focus on internet trolls instead of "in-real-life" bullies because the internet troll is a different creature, as it were. First of all, cruel posts that can be detrimental to one's social and occupational life never really go away. Where "in-real-life" bullying is over soon after it starts (even for an abusive written letter), internet posts can go on indefinitely and can always be revisited and reused by trolls.[1] Also, the internet provides more opportunity for trolls to create what Danielle Keats Citron calls "cyber mobs": large groups of trolls that get together to attack a single target.[2] Fat people have always had bullies, but the internet has allowed those bullies to become organized and legion.

Internet trolls are an often nebulous but sometimes well-organized group of people, and they have been studied and theorized. Typically, trolls shun communication in its interpersonal sense in favor of a complete annihilation of those who support or even marginally represent opposed viewpoints. Often, the opposed viewpoint is one that reflects a marginalized group's quest for acceptance and representation. Trolls are typically motivated by demoralizing such groups. Indeed, cruelty and a competitive quest for "lulz"—a pluralized play on the "Laugh Out Loud" acronym that suggests an inherent humor in attacking people on the internet—is a standard aspect of trolling, but the catalysts for trolling are a bit more complicated.

Primarily, we need to understand the "logic" of trolling; others have taken this on. Whitney Phillips's *This is Why We Can't Have Nice Things* aligns trolling with the Western affinity for agonistic rhetoric and a contemporary cultural logic that promotes one's right to be cruel.[3] She cites Socrates as a proto-troll (because, apparently, many trolls do, as well) and cites Arthur Schopenhauer as a godfather of trolling, who laid down a veritable but, perhaps, inadvertent "how-to" for trolling in *The Art of Controversy.*[4] When based on this understanding of Schopenhauer's work, the goal of trolling is not objective, agonistic debate for the sake of obtaining the truth. Instead, trolling's goal is a pseudo-objective, antagonistic debate for the sake of winning, whether right or wrong. When Schopenhauer discussed how to stave off interlocutors deemed "sophistic," today's trolls may take the side of his hypothetical negative interlocutor in hopes that their opponent has not read Schopenhauer or anyone else who has written about the proper detection of rhetorical fallacies. Schopenhauer has advice that can and has been taken by trolls for negative means. For example, Schopenhauer's advice to anger an opponent until he is too flustered to think clearly,[5] meant to defend against people hell-bent on winning instead of arriving at the truth, has been adopted by the latter's modern counterpart, trolls hell-bent on winning, as a way to fluster those in search of, or in defense of, the truth of a matter.

Even though their perceived ideological backing seems traditional and, according to Schopenhauer, practical, trolls take the fundamentals of Western thought and freedom to unhealthy extremes. Philosopher Richard Paul calls this "Sophistic Critical Thinking," which he defines as follows:

1. Thinking that meets epistemological demands insofar as they square with the vested interests of the thinker;
2. Skilled thinking that is heedless of assumptions, relevance, reasons, evidence, implications, and consistency only insofar as it is in the vested interest of the thinker to do so;
3. Skilled thinking that is motivated by vested interest, egocentrism, or ethnocentrism rather than by truth or objective reasonability.[6]

Trolling's *telos* is less virtuous in a traditional sense; it is the acquisition of power and the dismissal of truth and ethics. Hence, the rise of "alternative facts" and the demonization of empirically-based facts.

According to researchers, trolls know what they are doing. According to Phillips, one can conclude that a troll's ultimate motivation is to maintain the illusion of superiority at all costs. Most trolls partake of a phallocentric attitude—taken as mere logic and reason—that shuns relational and contextual thought[7] for such relational and contextual thought may come dangerously close to seeing the Other (racially, sexually, socioeconomically, physically, etc.) as an equal, and that cannot be tolerated. Thus trolling is an antidote to equality, political correctness (a tool used by champions of diversity for mutual respect that is infamously shunned by trolls) and insurance that those who enjoy hegemonic supremacy may continue to enjoy it. When it comes to Fat Acceptance, trolls are the "shock and awe" of hegemonic, anti-fat sentiment. So, when people do not fit the parameters of mainstream beauty standards, yet have the gall to carry themselves with pride, virtue, and a modicum of success, they are trolled.

One can define the seeds of "troll logic" as intense insecurity, fear of a loss of power, and a fear of vulnerability. Phillips conveys that much trolling is a kind of defense mechanism against a perceived angst and hopelessness of society.[8] That is, if thinness constitutes one's only "success" in life, but fat people are allowed to harbor self-pride and praise from others, the modicum of esteem derived from having a hegemonically acceptable body is substantially dissipated. Like many forms of discrimination and hate, anti-fat logic promotes an interpretation of the success of the "Other" as a threat to oneself.

Fearing the vulnerability that results from a loss of power and esteem may be the strongest motivator for trolling. In *Precarious Life: The Powers of Mourning and Violence*, Judith Butler cites vulnerability as the ultimate enemy of hegemony, for it fosters a sense of empathy and compassion for marginalized and oppressed people. But vulnerability has no place within troll logic; to feel vulnerable is to already have lost. Hegemony, *their* hegemony, must remain at all costs. Thus, vulnerability must be avoided at all costs.

To trolls, the Others of society are not even recognized as people, for doing so would induce a familiarity that, like vulnerability, would be detrimental to supremacist thinking. This is quite clear when it comes to anti-fat sentiment on the internet or in the media in general. (Think of images of fat bodies in news reports about obesity. Often, the image is from the neck down, erasing the head and, therefore, a sense of humanity in the subject.) Thus, as Butler explains, the Other is "derealized" and deemed "neither alive nor dead, but interminably spectral."[9] Trolls are especially cruel and relentless because they are not fighting a real, "living" entity, but something so "Other" as to not fit the contours of humanity. How much stronger is this phenomenon when considering the internet, where identities are relegated to mere non-contextualized content, reductive memes, and faceless words?

Thus, it is no surprise that the most vicious trolls are men carrying out a societal expectation to disassociate from their humanity with no consideration for context or the humanity involved in the particular subject matter.[10] Not surprisingly, being female is a major characteristic of troll victims. Danielle Keats Citron, in *Hate Crimes in Cyberspace* chronicles females victimized by sexist and sexually depraved trolls to the point of physical, emotional, and professional detriments. Sexual harassment is so deeply ingrained in American society, its amplified presence on the internet is no real mystery.[11] When one considers that the Fat Acceptance movement is predominantly female, the level of trolling is not surprising.

Trolls are a legitimate Discourse community, a "subculture" displaying "a set of unifying linguistic and behavioral practices."[12] Recalling James Gee's definition of a Discourse community as an "identity kit," one can see how trolls embody the "words, acts, values, beliefs, attitudes, social identities" that serve as "instructions on how to act, talk, and often write, so as to take on a particular social role that others will recognize"[13] Indeed, websites like 4chan served as incubators[14] where this Discourse was socially constructed by tech-savvy people disgusted by the onslaught of computer illiterates and activists pushing specific agendas.[15] A swath of "cyber-geeks" took on the roles of individual or collective pranksters using consistent terminology (e.g., lulz, cucks, etc.) and sharing a common motivation: indignant correction of those who either dilute their cyberculture or take themselves too seriously.

This dual nature of the troll's double raison d'etre—indignant correction of either those who defy cyber-geek sensibilities or those who take themselves too seriously—is important to a discussion of trolls and social activism. While researching and observing trolls, two distinct groups emerge. I call these groups "trickster trolls" and "hegemonic trolls."

Trickster trolls, motivated by the haphazard and seemingly random exploits of mythological and folkloric tricksters like Hermes or Brer Rabbit, respectively, attack for the sake of attacking. "I did it for the lulz" is a trolling axiom that fits them the most. The purpose is to flame others for the sole purpose of disruption and agitation of those deemed too self-righteous, despite their causes. Trickster trolls just want to watch the world burn; ideological indignation is not a major motivation. Trickster trolls despise what they see as exorbitantly sanctimonious, regarding "public displays of sentimentality, political conviction, and/or ideological rigidity" as impetuses for trolling.[16] (Ironically, trolls exist to troll other trolls who take their trolling too seriously, creating a vicious cycle.) Tricksters of mythology and folklore often exist for the very purpose of grounding those who may take themselves too seriously, forcing them to question their interpretations and certainties about the world.[17] Whitney writes: "The trolling mantra, 'Nothing should be taken seriously' suggests as much and functions both as a rallying cry and post hoc justification for trollish behavior. Trolls believe that, by wearing their hearts (or political affiliations, or sexual preferences, or other aspects of identity) on their sleeves, their targets are asking to be taught a lesson."[18]

Hegemonic trolls, however, are more directly didactic, motivated to perpetuate an ideology they deem correct and worthy of mass implementation, and correct those who think otherwise. Thus, when a person, especially an activist, comes along confidently and proudly exclaiming an opposing viewpoint, the trolls attack. Those who bring their social justice issues to the internet are attacked for assuming others share their sentiments; for that, they must be punished.[19] These trolls abide by what George Lakoff calls the "strict father" paradigm, which promotes dogma and the strict implementation of that dogma. Lakoff's description is worth quoting in full.

> In the strict father family, father knows best. He knows right from wrong and has the ultimate authority to make sure his children and his spouse do what he says, which is taken to be what is right. Many conservative spouses accept this worldview, uphold the father's authority, and are strict in those realms of family life that they are in charge of. When his children disobey, it is his moral duty to punish them painfully enough so that, to avoid punishment, they will obey him (do what is right) and not just do what feels good. Through physical discipline they are supposed to become disciplined, internally strong, and able to prosper in the external world. What if they don't prosper? That means they are not disciplined, and therefore cannot be moral, and so deserve their pover-

> ty. This reasoning shows up in conservative politics in which the poor are seen as lazy and undeserving, and the rich as deserving their wealth.[20]

The strict father paradigm produces an apt "identity kit" that is recognized in the behavior of many internet trolls. Hegemonic tricksters serve as an individual or a collective "strict parent," disciplining those who do not fall in line.

Both types of trolls exists in the general "anti-fat" online collective, but hegemonic tricksters tend to cause the most trouble, mainly because their viciousness is disguised as a mode of critical, pedagogical thinking far more focused than that of the trickster trolls. Hegemonic trolls perform as knowledgeable elites who know better, but are really out to railroad any agenda unlike their own, even if that agenda makes sense. Richard Paul's "Sophistic Critical Thinking," exemplifies this.

The main goal of hegemonic trolls is to push their agendas, even if they know their agendas are flawed. Purposeful fallacies of the logical, material, and psychological variety abound. The purpose in all of this is to push an agenda that helps them acquire power or maintain a power they already enjoy. Right or wrong, truth or falsehood, fact or fiction takes a back seat to possession of hegemonic power and a sense of superiority. One can see, then, how the display of pride and power from those who are not supposed to have it can set off the hegemonic troll. By extension, one can see why fat activists may be a favorite target.

ANTI-FAT TROLLS

In *Hate Crimes in Cyberspace,* Danielle Keats Citron tells the story of a young lady named Anna Mayer who wrote a pseudonymous blog on Fat Acceptance and other personal issues in 2008. Not much time passed before she was viciously harassed by bloggers hell-bent on ruining her self-esteem and her life. Not only did they send vicious and denigrating lies to prominent figures in her life (friends, professors, employers), but they let Anna know, in no uncertain terms, that they knew where she lived and encouraged people to visit her to perform sexually violent acts. As of 2014, she was still getting harassed by these trolls.[21]

These trolls attacked Anna because she was doing the unthinkable: living a positive life while fat. The fact that she was female also didn't help. Lakoff's description of the strict father extends to male superiority and, by extension, male chauvinism. In "Gendertrolling: Misogyny Adapts to New Media," Karla Mantilla writes that most victims of internet trolls are women (70%–76%)[22] and that their bodies and sexuality are often singled out.[23] When considering the predominately female and significantly genderqueer activists within the Fat Acceptance movement, their trolling was inevitable.

Defending oneself against trolls is a tricky ordeal. As we have seen, engaging with, or "feeding," the trolls only exacerbates their vitriol. Author Lindy West knows this all too well. In her book, *Shrill: Notes from a Loud Woman*, as well as her regular column in *The Guardian*, West, who often writes about being a woman of size, has given anecdotes and theorizations for why trolls troll. In her own experience, trolls are driven by motivations akin to those discussed above. However, she focuses more intently on the self-hatred she believes most internet trolls feel. Regarding one troll who apologized to her for his harassing behavior (a rare occurrence), people troll when they see someone who is not *supposed* to be happy enjoying his or her (most usually, her) life. That is, to a thin, white man who is miserable with his life, a fat woman's genuine happiness with her life is an affront—a reminder of his own failures. When a person who is supposed to be on top of the world is miserable, seeing someone who is supposed to be miserable exude genuine happiness can be disquieting.

West explains this during an interview on *The Sporkful*, a podcast about people's relationships with food. Talking of why thin people troll her the most, she says,

> just being a fat person who doesn't hate [yourself], there is this idea that you cheated or that you took something that wasn't yours. When people spend their whole lives participating in diet culture and pouring money and their whole lives into it, with the promise that at the end you feel happiness and fulfillment, and then a person like me declares that I deserve happiness and fulfillment now and then just goes and lives that way, people are like "Wait, I really invested a lot in this. What have I been doing with my life for the last twenty years? I could have just skipped to the finish line and been happy. . . . I think people are threatened by fat people having things that we construe as prizes for obedience and physical beauty.[24]

West provides a concise definition for trolls: people who punish those who don't deserve happiness. A happy fat person, in essence, "stole" that happiness. Sometimes, trolls feel like the happiness was stolen from them, specifically. A skinny troll may see a contented fat person as having taken what is rightfully his, similar to the old discriminatory complaint that a dominant groups' jobs are being "taken" by foreigners.

So is this a "trickster" troll or a hegemonic troll? Hegemony may be a driving justification—though not a driving motivation—for this troll's behavior. West was being shamed because she did not fit into socially acceptable categories of beauty or general worth. That is, she did not meet the criteria for American hegemony. So, to be clear, trolls can troll because, although hegemonic in many senses, they do not enjoy life as much as a marginal person who, by virtue of being marginal, does not deserve happiness. Trickster trolls, in theory, shun ideology and self-righteousness. Hegemonic trolls do so to the non-hegemonic, regardless of ideological stance.

This is seen most thoroughly when West debated comedian Jim Norton on the FX show, *Totally Biased.* West was asked to be on the show for her stance on rape jokes: they are never appropriate. Norton's stance, as is typical for televised debate shows, was the opposite: rape jokes are okay because they are just jokes.[25] The context of the debate was heavily in favor of Norton's stance; the crowd was full of comedy fans who bristled at the terms censorship, call-out culture, and even feminism,[26] so their willingness to ignore the logical fallacies from Norton were to be expected. Norton's fallacies—those of false equivalency, false dilemma, slippery slope, and false analogy—brought the debate away from the basic, and well-proven idea that language has an epistemic and empirical effect on society. Norton insisted that language did not have that much sway in society and that comedians and their fans take such off-color jokes as ways to think and ponder societal programs in a palatable way. He applied this to all comedians and their fans, exposing yet another fallacy, that of a hasty generalization.[27]

The fallout from the aired interview told all. West was bombarded by trolls who used her weight (and, therefore, her perceived unattractiveness) to silence her into irrelevancy. Some of their words are worth citing:

> You are really annoying. Don't worry no one would ever rape u. Worry about ur Health & the heart attack that's coming #uglycow.
> I love how the Bitch complaining about rape is the exact kind of Bitch that would never be raped. Bitch have you looked in the mirror.
> No one would want to rape that fat, disgusting mess.
> You're fat, ugly, and unfuckable. You don't have to worry about rape.
> There is no way a straight dude would fuck or even rape that ugly heifer. What an annoying cunt.
> Wouldn't the best ending be that Jim Norton rapes the fat girl.[28]

To her credit, West saw this as a victory, writing,

> They handed me a gift, I realized. A suffocating deluge of violent misogyny was how American comedy fans reacted to a woman suggesting that comedy might have a misogyny problem. They'd attempted to demonstrate that comedy, in general, doesn't have issues with women by threatening to rape and kill me, telling me I'm just bitter because I'm too fat to get raped . . . Their attempts to silence me made my point more effectively than any think piece or flawless debate performance ever could—they were churning out evidence as fast as they could type, hundreds of them working for me, for free.[29]

West's use of her trolls' vitriol had a positive effect, getting comedians—even Jim Norton—to condemn their behavior. According to West, the effect has lasted.

Although this is a success story, a larger problem still remains. Misogyny is very much a problem, and anti-fat sentiment exacerbates it. Hatred of fat bodies is clearly present in the trolls' comments, strongly suggesting that it is a favored tool in their general war on women. These trolls may have calmed down, but they calmed down when the men told them to. Although West's troll eventually came around and apologized, most do not. Apologies from trolls are rare and West still has several trolls to deal with. In fact, these several trolls often create organized forums from which trolling is actually planned and carried out. Sites like Anonymous and 4Chan have become infamous for housing such sites, but many abound. What is more, many are dedicated to specific ideas and specific people, including Fat Acceptance activists.

Ragen Chastain provides chilling examples of the aforementioned anti-fat trolls. Chastain, a fat woman who is well-known in the Fat Acceptance movement through her blog "Dances with Fat"[30] and "Ironfat"[31] (a blog chronicling her training for Iron Man races), is no stranger to organized trolls.

Some trolls have gone as far as creating their own sites to mock Chastain, like the blog "Dances with Facts," that claims, in no uncertain terms, that Ragen is dishonest and immoral. This site, which deals in what many in Fat Acceptance call concern trolling, done by "trolls who couch their trolling in healthism and ableism—insisting that they are only mistreating fat people because [they] are unhealthy or because of the money we cost the healthcare system,"[32] decided to attack Chastain, specifically, as opposed to the organization that provides the foundation of Chastains thoughts on weight and health: the Association for Size Diversity and Health, an organization of which the "Dances with Facts" coordinators are well aware.

Why did this site and sites like it focus on one individual instead of the source of that individual's beliefs? Why did the site not specifically attack Fat Acceptance professionals from a variety of fields—from healthcare to law and academia—instead of focusing on one particular person? One could conclude that "Dances with Facts," did not discern Chastain as having the ethos to either know what she is talking about or have the confidence and positivity she exudes on her blogs. Though the site claims to abhor negative treatment toward fat people, it specifically goes after Chastain for reasons both related and unrelated to the correlation of fat and health. It reads that the site's purpose is to "call into question [Chastain's] expertise on the science of obesity, her history of dishonest crowdfunding and solicitation of donations, the accuracy of her claims about a wide variety of subjects such as her athletics and the 'harassment' she faces, and most importantly her profound lack of integrity."[33] The fact that Chastain sites sources and the fact that the other claims are unfounded suggest such "concern" trolling is a subcategory of hegemonic trolling.

In an interview, Chastain elaborated on the possible motivations of her anti-fat trolls, stating "I think that it's a classic reaction to self-hate and self-loathing and a desperate need for community among people who are emotionally stunted. In fat hate sites they are able to find the community that they are so desperate for, organized around putting others down in a way that makes them feel better than somebody, and powerful."[34] Sites like "Dances With Facts" fit this description. Most trolls tend to participate in group trolling and can find a variety of niches on the internet, but hegemonic trolls may get the most out of their group solidarity. In a group, a sense of belonging both satiates and motivates its members.

Trolls, especially hegemonic trolls, are no different. Chastain elaborates on her experience with such troll "armies":

> My trolls are quite organized (the largest forum dedicated to hating me that I'm aware of has 4,000 people, there are a number of others, the forums are where the lies and half-truths about me are formulated and perfected, and the hatred of me is clear and plain. Then they have websites that are created to look legitimate that they use to try to disrupt my life and work by, for example, e-mailing anyone who partners with me with a list of lies about me (everything from the suggestion that I cheat at races to the suggestion that I'm an animal abuser). The attacks on my personally tend to be coordinated and personal (ie: a troll will discover a quote I gave a small town paper in third grade and I'll receive a couple hundred e-mails about it).[35]

If these tactics seem too petty to fit into the hegemonic category of trolls, they still pack a hegemonic punch. Often, members of troll groups join for the ideology—or even for the opportunity to troll—while letting the leaders be the spokespeople. Chastain confirms this in her interview: "In my experience it seems that there are a few trolls operating under this description [of hegemonic troll], and then many others who simply follow them, performing the role of zealots—believing anything that the leaders say, however improbable or ridiculous, and boosting their signal via typical trolling techniques."[36]

So, troll armies, like most armies, are equipped with their generals and their foot soldiers, leaders, and followers. Thus, much trolling of fat activists may be motivated by hegemonic ideals that are categorically anti-fat, but end in ways meant not to simply disprove an ideology, but destroy the agents of that ideology. In fact, destroying the agents of a marginal ideology is more important to trolls than actually disproving an ideology; silencing someone is easier than debating someone. Again, Chastain has lived this.

> A few years ago my trolls found out that my brother had died by suicide. Out of the blue I received hundreds of e-mails and blog comments asking if my brother killed himself because I was his sister and/or suggesting that I should do as he had done.

> I was giving two paid talks at a college and when their protest of my first talk was completely unsuccessful they set off the fire alarm trying to get my second talk cancelled.
>
> After receiving e-mails threatening to drown me in the swim of my half IRONMAN, one of them found me in line at the start (which meant picking me out of nearly 2,000 athletes all wearing the same wetsuit and swim cap) called me by name and then asked "What did Reddit say about you this morning?" I found out later that others had been there trying to get as close as possible to my family and me in order to take video and pictures to post to a hate site (which preemptively threatened to sue me if I posted pictures of them).[37]

The most telling aspect of these troll armies is that their victims share one thing: singularity. Most trolling events involve several people attacking a single person. Instead of attacking an ideology, which would make them another iteration of the social justice warrior, they let a single person personify that ideology. What this says about troll armies of either the hegemonic or the trickster variety is not as important as what it implies about strategies for dealing with trolls.

Here is where we return to the mechanisms of Structuration and activism. Institutional backing is a strong tool (weapon) against troll armies. Institutionalization suggests hegemony. What's more, institutions are much harder to silence than normal individuals. Government protection, popularized symbolism, and ideological legitimacy help solidify and justify one's place in the world. Fat Activism has certainly been buttressed by these things. Also, alignment—joining forces with already established institutions—does much to bring marginalized people into protected space where they are not sitting ducks for trolls. There is power in numbers, a collective yell is harder to shut down than a single whisper.

Along with *Shrill,* Lindy West is media ubiquity. She is fortunate enough to write for *GQ* and *The Guardian*, respected publications read by millions in print and electronic form. She is the founder and editor of *I Believe You/It's Not Your Fault*, an advice blog for teenagers. She has appeared on stage, on television, and on radio and podcasts discussing Fat Acceptance, internet trolls, and feminism. She was even included in *Cosmopolitan*'s "Internet's Most Fascinating of 2015." Clearly, West has made the best of a variety of media that is generally accepted in hegemonic spaces. Couching alternative viewpoints like Fat Acceptance in hegemonic Discourses of culture and lifestyle seems to be a worthwhile alignment. She is becoming a well-known figure in a variety of social and professional circles.

Ragen Chastain is the editor of a two-volume collection of essays titled *The Politics of Size: Perspectives from the Fat Acceptance Movement.* This mix of scholarly and non-scholarly essays speaks to various parts of Fat Acceptance, including intersectionality, physical and mental health, fitness, and workplace issues. When taking her public speaking and personal branding into consideration, Chastain has successfully maneuvered in both Signification and Domination, at least. Regarding Domination, she successfully accomplished this aspect of Structuration by effectively aligning herself with academic and healthcare professionals.

The only thing that seems to weaken trolls are numbers and power. (One could say that the acquisition of group solidarity and power is a main impetus for trolling, in the first place.) West and Chastain do wonderful jobs modeling successful ways to gain numbers and power, but the fight is far from over. Perhaps the ultimate tool of hegemony is not just ideological backing, but metanarrative backing. That is, a powerful ideology is always backed by an implicit story that adequately sells that ideology. Does Fat Acceptance have such a story?

NOTES

1. Danielle Keats Citron, *Hate Crimes in Cyberspace* (Cambridge, MA: Harvard University Press, 2014), 4.
2. Ibid., 5.
3. Whitney Phillips, *This is Why We Can't Have Nice Things* (Cambridge, MA: MIT Press, 2015), 118.
4. Ibid., 124–126.
5. Arthur Schopenhauer, *The Art of Controversy*, E-book, Loc 332.
6. Richard Paul, "Critical Thinking in North America," *Critical Thinking: What Every Person Needs to Survive in a Rapidly Changing World*, (Tomales, CA: Foundation for Critical Thinking, 2012), 47.
7. Phillips, 125–126.
8. Ibid., 122–212.
9. Judith Butler, *Precarious Life: The Powers of Mourning and Violence*, (New York: Verso, 2004), 33.
10. Ibid, 34–36.
11. Danielle Keats Citron, *Hate Crimes in Cyberspace* (Cambridge, MA: Harvard University Press, 2014), 254.
12. Philips, 17.
13. James Gee, *Social Linguistics and Literacies: Ideology and Discourses* (Bristol, PA: The Falmer Press, 1990), 142.
14. Philips, 20.
15. E. Gabriella Coleman, "Phreaks, Hackers, and Trolls: The Politics of Transgression and Spectacle." In *The Social Media Reader*, edited by Mandiberg Michael, 113 (New York: NYU Press, 2012), http://www.jstor.org.ezproxy.ycp.edu:8000/stable/j.ctt16gzq5m.12.
16. Philips, 25.
17. Bradley John Monsma. "'Active Readers . . . Observe Tricksters': Trickster Texts and Cross-Cultural Reading." *Modern Language Studies* 26, no. 4 (1996): 84. doi:10.2307/3195326.
18. Philips, 25.
19. Ibid.
20. George Lakoff, "Understanding Trump," *George Lakoff.* Accessed Aug. 3 2017. https://georgelakoff.com/2016/07/23/understanding-trump-2/.
21. Citron, 1–3.
22. Ibid., 13–14.
23. Karla Mantilla, "Gendertrolling: Misogyny Adapts to New Media." *Feminist Studies* 39, no. 2 (2013): 563–570. http://www.jstor.org.ezproxy.ycp.edu:8000/stable/23719068 .

24. "How to Be Fat," *The Sporkful*, accessed July 28, 2017, http://www.sporkful.com/how-to-be-fat-with-lindy-west/.
25. Lindy West, *Shrill: Notes from a Loud Woman*, (New York: Hachette Books, 2016), 182–194.
26. Ibid., 182.
27. Ibid., 190.
28. Ibid., 196–201.
29. Ibid., 203.
30. Ragen Chastain, *Dances with Fat*, accessed August 3, 2017, https://danceswithfat.wordpress.com/blog/.
31. Ragen Chastain, *Ironfat*, accessed August 3, 2017, https://ironfatblog.wordpress.com/.
32. Ragen Chastain (fat activist) interviewed by Erec Smith, email, July 26, 2017.
33. "Dances with Facts," accessed August 3, 2017, https://truthaboutragen.wordpress.com/.
34. Chastain, interview.
35. Ibid.
36. Ibid.
37. Ibid.

Chapter Five

The Power of Narrative in Fat Acceptance

One would be hard-pressed to find a relatively well-read person, or an avid movie-goer, or a lover of theater who would deny the power of storytelling, outright. Often, to listen to one's story is to, at least inadvertently, see some part of yourself in him or her. Stories induce a more visceral understanding of a subject for most. To be shown and not told constructs a more relaxed learning environment where information is meant to be retained through a kind of cathexis as opposed to a rote memory. It is fair to say that story has been a most holistic form of pedagogy at least since Homer recited the *Illiad*.

However, in some circles, many considered erudite in nature, people would shun "the story" as a mode of intellectual thought and didacticism. This suggests that, perhaps, those of low intellectual capability need their information fed to them via narrative, but "real" thought follows, to some degree, a scientific method or pertains to the fundamentals of a logocentric, academic Discourse. Thus, story as a pedagogy or epistemology is not taken seriously.

That being said, if one is trying to revise an ideology they deem both misinformed and oppressive, one would do well to realize that ideologies spread most effectively via narrative—either a localized narrative of anecdotal character or a more global metanarrative perpetuated by various media. Perhaps a culture of power devised hegemonic ideology in more "academic" ways, but the ideologies took hold en masse via stories of some form. Thus, to combat belief-systems brought on by narrative, one may do well to construct a counter-narrative.

One can look at Giddens's Structuration and notice how the power of story feeds into Signification, Legitimation, and Dominance. One can see how stories can create "morals" that result in self-pride and group pride.

From the standpoint of a marginal social activist, like a fat activist, the power of story—or, in a more academic context, as with Fat Studies scholars, the power of autoethnography—is a (if not *the*) primary rhetorical strategy. Of course, in order for storytelling to work, it has to act locally *and* globally. I agree that this is happening often on the local level, but on a global level, as with metanarrative, the Fat Studies movement may still be in its beginning stages.

LOCAL STORYTELLING

When I talk about the local in storytelling as a mode of teaching, thinking, and knowing, I mean anecdotal experiences that speak to the struggles and triumphs of one or a group of people in a relatively localized context. Relaying a personal experience is a form of local storytelling; that experience gives insight into the nature of a struggle and puts a face to one who is affected by it. Such stories abound in the form of books, blogs, interviews, and video.

Marie Southard Ospina is a journalist, self-proclaimed Fat Acceptance activist and storyteller. Ospina puts activism and storytelling together in a video titled "Redefining Fat"[1] produced by StylelikeU, a website dedicated to "radical self-acceptance" for their "What's Underneath" series.[2] One can already glean a story about Fat Acceptance and pride in the name of positive identity politics, but Ospina's storytelling and performance, itself, lends a power to these ideas that cannot be accomplished by polemical rhetoric.

Ospina not only tells a story of overcoming body shame as a fat woman, but does so while intermittently removing pieces of clothing until she is in her underwear. Thus, Ospina supplements an oral story about her triumph over fat stigma with the visual task of showing her stigmatized body for all to see. To be fair, clothing removal is requisite for participating in the "What's Underneath" series, but that, too, speaks to the power of oral and visual storytelling.

Opsina's story moves along the lines of a hero's journey on an epic scale, but also like Cinderella on the fairy tale scale. This overlap with two narrative journeys with proven cultural influence strengthens both Ospina and the power of her story. It moves her from autobiographical narrator to protagonist fighting antagonistic forces.

As the main character, Ospina starts out *in medias res*, discussing how she began concealing her body at a young age but now confronts it to both enhance self-esteem and battle societal stigma. She backtracks to discuss how family and schoolmates consistently bombarded her with criticisms and insults about her weight. This ill treatment resulted in ill health; she developed an eating disorder as a teenager. However, what got her through those tough years and would shape her currently healthy life was journaling and experiencing a world where body shaming was outside hegemonic normality. Her writing—the tool she used to escape a fat-shaming world and express her feelings—would become her livelihood and a ticket to professional success. A study abroad program in Spain would show her that fat stigma was not a natural occurrence but a social construct crafted by aesthetically restricted, thin-obsessed (often disguised as health-obsessed) culture. This trip to Spain is where she would find a romantic partner, a thin British man, who would remain her partner long afterward. From this experience, the Marie Southard Ospina we know—the prolific writer and size activist—was born.

One can see the classic narrative of a downtrodden protagonist struggling with the abuses and constraints of her environment, who discovers the tools and people who would help her triumph over a collective and ideological enemy. Ospina's story seems to parallel many stories told by fat activists across the United States and England. Thus, a narrative of triumph or of a phoenix rising from the ashes to advocate for oneself and others seems to be the primary narrative of Fat Activism as a movement of pride and identity. Again, the visual component of this particular telling cannot be dismissed. Ospina's protagonist triumphs within a plot that is partly told and partly shown. She *vocalizes* a journey to self-acceptance, but she *shows* that she has arrived at her destination. This combination of oral and visual rhetoric tells a powerful story that can go far toward enhancing self and group pride.

GLOBAL STORYTELLING

The metanarrative is something a bit more complicated. This grand story does not simply motivate its audience to believe certain things or to behave in certain ways; it legitimizes those beliefs and behaviors on a societal scale. One could say that the true protagonist in a metanarrative is the ideology it is meant to illustrate and perpetuate. Thus, any social movement would do well to establish one of its own. Jonathan Smucker insists that narrative, constructed properly, is the key to activist-induced social change and the instillation of a belief system. Even his thoughts on interpersonal communication come into play; its unapologetic pragmatism may also be a key aspect of his narrative activism.

Let's take, for instance, his concept of narrative attack and narrative insurgency. Narrative attack is not an attack on another's stance through the use of narrative. It is the tendency to attack another's metanarrative, that is, another's entire belief system, straight away. Smucker gives the example of a climate change denier who cites creationism as the source of his belief. Attacking creationism, something this person probably holds dear, will do more harm than good, prompting him or her to shut down.[3] However, the act of narrative insurgency meets the person where he or she is by offering what

Smucker calls "ally beliefs": beliefs that already exist within a belief system that can be reinforced to enhance empathy and relationality. Returning to the hypothetical creationist, Smucker would suggest the biblical imperative that humans must respect and take care of God's creation, regardless of climate change's legitimacy.[4]

How might this look within the Fat Acceptance movement? I know that when people diagnose fat people as "unhealthy" just by appearance, my first desire is to embark on a narrative attack, discussing how many medical assumptions about the correlation of size and health are often erroneous or inconclusive. This can—indeed, it has—created immediate pushback, especially from those who would identify with their thin or relatively thin bodies. However, if I were to abide by narrative insurgence, perhaps I would find common ground with the person's affinity for a healthy lifestyle. I may bring up Kelly Bliss, *Health At Every Size®* ideology, or Ragen Chastain's chronicled workout regimen to say that fat people do appreciate health regardless of how they may look.

This may come off as kowtowing, and it would be if the act were to stop there. This tactic is just that: a tactic; one step of many toward Fat Acceptance. As Smucker writes, "Narrative insurgents don't reject problematic narratives wholesale, but instead identify and distinguish between those components of a narrative that are *allied, hostile*, or *neutral* to our cause. We embrace as much of a cultural narrative as possible—the allied and neutral components—and use this as a foundation for our organizing efforts with and within the given community."[5] Again, this is more pragmatic and less comfortable to some degree. As a black man, I find it difficult to try to listen to and find commonality with white supremacists or even "casual" racists. However, to think pragmatically is to do what may be most efficient and expedient to one's cause. The road to hegemony starts with short and, sometimes, painful steps.

This, however, may be the only way to accomplish change through metanarrative: end or heavily revise the old metanarrative. Many attempts at working with others are thwarted by reminding people of already established metanarratives and, especially, their accompanying stereotypes. When fat people reach out to explain to authority figures in logical and clear ways that health correlations are not solid and laziness is not a common trait among them, the stereotype of "unintelligent," "lazy," and, therefore, "untrustworthy," fat people rears its head. The best way to combat this may be to find common ground so ingrained in preexisting modes of virtue that a new "we" comes into shape.[6]

"We," here, is related to be what Kenneth Burke refers to as a terministic screen, a filter into society where certain ideas and values are selected while others are deflected.[7] That is, every instance of a pro-fat metanarrative must lay on a foundation of social unification; a commonality to be effectively written and incorporated. Smucker, suggesting a similar idea, presents the difference between a terministic screen of "we" and one of "they." Regarding a screen of "we," he writes, "As a society, we must have law and order." Regarding "they," he writes, "They're a bunch of outside agitators."[8] One can easily see the differences, the benefits and detriments of the screens, respectively. Thus, this narrative has to maintain a terministic screen of holistic unity, and this narrative must be systemic in all we do, throughout all aspects of Structuration, through aligning, even through dealing with trolls and the harshest of anti-fat bullies. This is how we create not just a metanarrative, but a corresponding Discourse of Fat Acceptance. In Gee's definition we see an "identity kit"[9] to go along with the "we" oriented metanarrative. Every story needs a protagonist, and that protagonist has an identity that is unique yet resonates with others with which she/he forms a "we."

All this is a tall order, but Smucker has a formula for creating a terministic screen and Discourse (behavior, values, words, etc.). He provides a "worksheet" titled "Anatomy of a Political Narrative," to help activists formulate a we-oriented and Discourse-building metanarrative.[10] My following application of Fat Acceptance to this narrative template is by no means prescriptive. (I cannot emphasize that enough.) I should say, however, that what I find missing from Smucker's conception of metanarrative is the "march of history" concept. Smucker focuses on the idea of metanarratives as a kind of collective visionary frame, but he neglects—or ignores—the historical development of a metanarrative as dialectical. That is, a current metanarrative is thought to be the result of a synthesis of previous ideologies throughout history.

I think Smucker ignores this aspect of metanarrative because, like postmodernists, he sees metanarrative as distinctly fictional, arbitrary fabrications put together by hegemonic forces that act as historical curators, choosing the aspects of Discourse to be displayed as one sociological unit. The fictional nature of metanarrative, however, does not negate its value. Stories are still needed to create and perpetuate metanarratives, even if they are essentially "make believe." Smucker writes that although postmodernism's deconstruction of metanarrative as arbitrary fiction is correct from an analytical standpoint[11] it is a mistake to stop there. Once an oppressive metanarrative is deflated, something must take its place, for metanarratives, though fictional, are an ontological necessity. If activists are to enter or revise hegemony, they must not only topple that hegemony; they must fabricate one of their own it its polace.[12]

Thus, the march of history aspect of metanarrative is less important than the contemporary necessity to build one, according to Smucker. However, I think it is important to emphasize that metanarratives tend to take hold because they are sold as natural consequences of history. Metanarratives are constructed as ideology that inevitably occurred from the march of history.

So, Smucker neglects to mention a key rule when constructing a metanarrative: Take context into consideration. The story has to make sense as a reasonable effect to the cause that is history or, at least, a relatively present moment of departure. William James's pragmatism necessitates a consideration of past and current attitudes when affecting change. If one strays too far from societal norms, the change is too abrupt to be adopted. However, if that change still maintains most of those norms, the change is more palatable. That is, true change happens slowly. A metanarrative meant to induce change must still look familiar to its subjects. To take some creative license with one of Smucker's concepts, this strategy may be recognized as *meta*narrative insurgency.

THE GRAND NARRATIVE OF FAT ACCEPTANCE

In a chapter titled "The 'We' in Politics," Smucker discusses how the Center for Story-Based Strategy motivated his social justice organization, "Beyond the Choir," to use a narrative outline to both understand the hegemonic narrative and their own. The outline consists of the following prompts:

Who is the we?
Who is the other?
Who are the protagonists
Who are the villains? What are the threats?
What is the conflict?
Emotions?
Symbols and images?
Assumptions?
Vulnerabilities?
Deadwood?[13]

Based on the observations in this book, I have filled in the outline with *a* take on the Fat Acceptance metanarrative. I cannot emphasize enough the use of the indefinite article here; this is merely one take on the narrative displayed as an example of how this outline can be used as a foundational, motivational, and strategic tool for the movement.

Who is the we?

The "we" in the Fat Acceptance movement consists of fat activists or scholars and their allies. Most often, the fat activists are, themselves, fat and, therefore, familiar with the detriments of fat stigma from both individuals and society, at large. Other than allies—who I define as people working for Fat Acceptance who have not dealt with fat shaming—the bulk of this "we" consists of those who not only want to fight fat stigma, but keenly know how it feels to be negatively affected by such stigma. The "we" shares both the pain of fat stigma as well as the motivation and knowledge to combat it.

Who is the other?

The other is a diverse group that consists of people who share anti-fat sentiment for (apparently) several different reasons; aesthetics, health-based concerns, economics, weight-loss industry interests, and moral implications come to mind. Ultimately, it is believed that fat bodies are a literal and figurative disease that must be staved off for the overall well-being of society. Thus, cruelty toward fat people is justified as a necessary tactic.

Who are the protagonists?

Unlike the "Who is the we?" question, "Who are the protagonists?" asks who the audience (society at large) finds relational, as well. Based on common conceptions of effective story and plot, the "hero" has a particular ethos: he or she is a likeable person who must overcome a challenge in a way that produces both benefit and personal growth. I am reminded of the quasi-satirical article "The 12 Good Fatty Archetypes" written by Stacy Bias, which elaborates upon several archetypal subject positions held by fat people.[14] Of course, these archetypes derive from the hegemonic narrative that is being combatted, but for strategic purposes, this question necessitates an insurgent narrative that uses common ground as a starting point toward moving people along the (hero's) journey to Fat Acceptance.

Bias's archetypes—The Good Fatty, the Work-in-Progress, the Mama Hen, etc.—express ways in which fat bodies are shamed the least. Of course, the characteristic of being misunderstood by a misguided (not necessarily evil—remember the impetus for an insurgent narrative) populace is imperative as well. With all these considerations presented, Bias's caveat is important: "Where the 'Good Fatty' becomes problematic is when it's used as a justification for social legitimacy—when it says 'I deserve to be seen as valuable because (insert "good fatty" stereotype here).' We *all* deserve to be seen as valuable, wherever we're at in our individual journeys with our bodies, our self-esteem, and our politics."[15] For our purposes, the operative term in Bias's caveat is "individual journey"; no one should feel like they must abide by these archetypes to be accepted by society. However, when crafting an effective metanarrative, creating a hero that seems to reflect one of these archetypes may be rhetorically effective.

Who are the villains? What are the threats?

The villains are a diverse collective. Unlike the Other, however, the villain is necessarily cruel and oppressive. These are the trolls and the celebrity designers who do not want fat people wearing their clothes or, which is often the case, do not even make clothes beyond a certain size. These are the bullies who use thinness as a blatant mode of supremacy. On a more speculative note, these are medical professionals who automatically diagnose fat people as unhealthy without going through the proper steps to come to that conclusion.

What is the conflict?

To be more specific, Smucker asks, "How is the conflict framed in order to appeal to the audience's values (i.e., to win the audience's sympathy)?"[16] This may seem obvious based on answers to previous questions, but perhaps we can see this in two ways: the conflict is either a matter of morality (we should not be cruel to people of size) or a matter of knowledge (we do not have the proper knowledge to label fat bodies based on beliefs about health and fitness). Ideally, for a metanarrative of Fat Acceptance, both aspects can be creatively combined to create a grand conflict to be resolved.

Emotions

This is where pathos comes in: how do we want the societal audience to feel about collective protagonists? Do we want the audience to be angry about the protagonist's plight? Do we want them to feel empathy? Anger? Whatever emotion or emotions are chosen, the goal should be to promote commonality and be relational. Again, Smucker's description of an insurgent narrative comes to play in that we must gauge the audience and determine which emotion will be most effective.

Symbols and images

Here, we come back to Signification as an important mode of Giddens's Structuration. For constructing a metanarrative, we must utilize symbols already appreciated by the audience as well as those appropriated and revised by fat activists. Smucker brings up the importance of symbols often; symbols need not become veritable "mascots" of the movement, but their familiarity and invocation of a shared lifestyle are imperative. Besides the iconic symbols discussed in chapter 2, more common images of fat people enjoying life in ways they are not supposed to deserve function well, here. Pictures of confident and happy models like Tess Holiday, glamorous entertainers like Gabriel Sidibe and Adele, athletes like Prince Fielder, and others fit the bill, presenting fat people as happy, successful, and even enviable.

Assumptions

What is the warrant in this story? That is, what must the audience already believe? Again, the answer to that question is strongly implied in the previous answers, but articulating this is important to constructing an effective narrative. As a conceptual overlap with the "Symbols and Images" prompt, this belief must be both integral to the audience's society and beneficial to the goals of the protagonist. The concept of "life, liberty, and the pursuit of happiness," could be such a belief; this justifies the triumphant attitude of the protagonist to an audience who firmly embraces the same concept.

Vulnerabilities

Here, the crafters of the metanarrative need to be honest and objective about vulnerabilities, that is, places most susceptible to scrutiny. For example, some medical assumptions are not wrong, but "inconclusive." Thus, charging health-inspired anti-fat agents with deception may not be accurate at all times. Much anti-fat sentiment is put out by people who hold the proper medical or scientific ethos for their conclusions, even if those conclusions were not arrived at in strictly scientific ways, so combatting them can be difficult.

Deadwood

What aspects are unnecessary or "beside the point." Often, people cite romantic couples involving a thin person (typically male) and a fat person (typically female) to justify fat bodies. These instances could be construed as "beside the point," in that the condition and looks of one's lover need not dictate societal acceptance; regardless of whom one dates, the aforementioned issues and goals of the Fat Acceptance movement do not change. (A thin male could be used as a "symbol or image," but, possibly, this could do more harm than good, even from an insurgent narrative strategy: such a symbol smacks of the "savior" motif and takes power away from the protagonist.)

How this metanarrative pans out depends on how we combine these answers and considerations into a story about Fat Acceptance. A literal story, like that of Ospina, need not come to fruition. Each of the ten prompts can be perpetuated until society starts to put together the story, itself. This is a tall order, and the "we" from prompt one is already quite diligent in working toward it. Again, the responses to these prompts are just my subjective ideas. Smucker suggests using these prompts in workshops and conferences to create a consensus, more or less, of how a metanarrative should play out. I only provide my take as a model for doing so based on my observations and my concerns for Fat Acceptance.

I should end this chapter and book by discussing the concept of insurgent narrative and pragmatism. In an essay I wrote for the anthology *The Politics of Size*, I assert that the issues of race and ethnicity within the Fat Acceptance movement must be dealt with, but in ways prompted by the concept of pragmatism: a strategic use of contingent practical elements. In line with insurgent narrative, I saw how white faces are—not *should be*—the mainstream faces of the movement and that we should somehow find a way to utilize this fact to move toward more diversity in Fat Acceptance.[17] Many activists read my words as saying that people of color should take a back seat to white activists until things change. This could not be farther from my point.

As Smucker articulates, movements built for group esteem are very important, but not the final step toward societal Fat Acceptance. Strategic considerations beyond group morale must be put forward and utilized. Based on this consideration, I provide the above responses to the narrative prompts.

NOTES

1. Marie Southard Ospina, "Redefining Fat," *StyleLikeU*, accessed 26 Sept. 2017, https://www.youtube.com/watch?v=YwF5D0UPEbo.
2. "What's Underneath," *StyleLikeU*, accessed 26 Sept. 2017, http://stylelikeu.com/category/the-whats-underneath-project-2/.
3. Jonathan Smucker, *Hegemony How-To: A Roadmap for Radicals*, (Chico, CA: AK Press, 2017), 192.
4. Ibid., 192.
5. Ibid., 193.
6. Ibid., 216–218.
7. Kenneth Burke, *Language As Symbolic Action* (Berkeley: University of California Press, 1966).
8. Smucker, 224.
9. James Paul Gee, *Social Linguistics and Literacies: Ideology and Discourses* (Bristol, PA: The Falmer Press, 1990), 142.
10. Ibid., 230–231.
11. Ibid., 219.
12. Ibid., 220–222.
13. Ibid., 230–231.
14. Stacy Bias, "The 12 Good Fatty Archetypes," accessed 26 Sept. 2017, http://stacybias.net/2014/06/12-good-fatty-archetypes/.
15. Ibid.
16. Smucker, 231.
17. Erec Smith, "The Pragmatic Attitude in Fat Acceptance: Race and Rhetoric in the Fat Acceptance Movement," (Santa Barbara, CA: Praeger Press, 2015).

Conclusion

Seeing how Giddens's Structuration has shaped Fat Activism strongly suggests that progress toward hegemony is an interdependent endeavor. Signification, Domination, and Legitimation each depend on a team effort consisting of different agents, institutions, symbols, and commonplaces. They also depend on the preestablished nature of these things. Structuration must begin, then, by latching on to preexisting structures and creating new outgrowths or renderings of these structures that do not immediately shift paradigms but alter paradigms enough to authenticate new ideas, agents, and activities.

William James's concept of pragmatism comes into play, here. Structuration, as just described, is an inherently gradual mode of activism. According to James, the gradual nature of structuration is not a choice but a result of the very nature of change. In his essay "What Pragmatism Means," James writes

> Our minds thus grow in spots; and like grease-spots, the spots spread. But we let them spread as little as possible: we keep unaltered as much of our old knowledge, as many of our old prejudices and beliefs, as we can. We patch and tinker more than we renew. The novelty soaks in; it stains the ancient mass; but it is also tinged by what absorbs it. Our past apperceives and co-operates; and in the new equilibrium in which each step forward in the process of learning terminates, it happens relatively seldom that the new fact is added raw. More usually it is embedded cooked, as one might say, or stewed down in the sauce of the old. . . . New truths thus are resultants of new experiences and of old truths combined and mutually modifying one another. [1]

James is talking mostly of the individual or humanity as sentient beings, but the connection to societal structures is easy to see. I would extend James's theory on the pragmatic nature of change by saying that certain factions of society need to be infiltrated to certain degrees.

Compare James's theory on pragmatic change with Smucker's "narrative insurgency" and my own arguments in "The Pragmatic Attitude in Fat Activism," and we see a tactical necessity for using old symbols and beliefs to birth social change. Structuration, too, can morph into the new instead of being catastrophically disrupted or deconstructed in order to build anew. Attaching an addition to an already established house may be more efficient than demolishing a structure to build another in its place. Each aspect of Structuration is a gradual outgrowth of a common mode of interpretation (Signification) a common idea of what necessitates legal protection (Legitimation) and common institutional ideologies (Domination).

In "The Pragmatic Attitude in Fat Activism: Race and Rhetoric in the Acceptance Movement," I discuss the need to acknowledge this change "within" the Fat Acceptance movement regarding racial diversity. I argued that a pragmatic take must reorganize the generally discriminatory nature of America and work as an outgrowth to change the racial dynamics within the movement. If minority status is already problematic, its synthesis with fat status could create a bigger challenge. The gradual growth of Fat Studies—with its interdisciplinary nature—may suggest an even more gradual growth of diversity within the movement.[2]

As I mentioned at the end of chapter 5, my thesis offended many fat activists, white and people of color, alike. They read my essay as a justification of the neglect of minority concerns. This was not the case. Pragmatic strategy does not mean diversity within the Fat Acceptance movement cannot co-manifest with the general Acceptance of Fat Activism by society. I merely argued that pragmatism would mean that audiences have to be gauged and engaged, accordingly. I think this warrants repeating. In essence, pragmatic strategy must be *kairotic*, that is, contingent on the dictates of a particular situation; it must be interdependent on what a context provides. Interpellations must be taken seriously while still being altered and played with, as much as the situation will allow without sacrificing progress. The general point is that activists need a combination of Structuration and pragmatism to create and maintain change.

I believe this is a rhetorical issue. In ways tried and true to general topic of rhetorical invention (coming up with what to articulate and how to articulate it), activists reshape common modes of understanding (what are called "topoi" in rhetorical theory) like comparison, definition, and cause and effect relationships in their favor. Definition as a mode of understanding may be most salient, here. This mode, articulated as a genus/species understanding of things, helps establish foundation concepts on which thought and behaviors depend. Regarding definition's relationship to Signification, the "genus" of beauty or virtue is packaged with the "species" of fat bodies and fat people, exuding a kind of *kalos kai agathos*: effective confluence of beauty and virtue. Further, the context (genus) of beauty filled with the image of fat bodies (species)—lingerie ads, Adipositivity, *Volup2* magazine, and so forth—help redefine beauty. The perpetuation of definition as a common mode of understanding in rhetorical invention helps smooth transitions into the mainstream.

The topic of definition applies to the other aspects of Structuraiton, as well. Domination provides the genus of identity studies (perhaps under the "kingdom" of academia, to extend the biology analogy) with the species of Fat Studies to accompany other academic fields and sub-fields. Following the lead and *raison d'etre* of other fields like gender studies or African American studies—emulation, to some degree—is key to the pragmatic transition into academia. Similarly, the genus of equal rights activism can harbor specific groups. Fat activists, emulating others, ease into this genus. Healthcare concerns may actually be a subspecies of sorts; equal rights easily extend to equal medical rights. Definition's relationship to Legitimation may be exemplified best through the American Creed. "Life, Liberty, and the pursuit of Happiness" is not supposed to be denied to people based on body size. Once fat is redefined as something not inherently ignoble, discrimination based on fat may be seen as unethical and un-American. Legal protections would be soon to follow.

This brings us to the very term "fat" and its redefinition. Structuration comes together to redefine the term "fat." In fact, fat as a dominate "God" term, has given birth to a Discourse that both shares the values, beliefs, and behaviors of hegemonic Discourses but adds terminology and behavior that creates a distinct fat Discourse. James Gee's definition of Discourse is worth revisiting. According to Gee,

> A Discourse with a capital "D" is composed of distinctive ways of speaking/listening and often, too, writing/reading coupled with distinctive ways of acting, interacting, valuing, feeling, dressing, thinking, believing, with other people and with various objects, tools, and technologies, so as to enact specific socially recognizable identities engaged in specific socially recognizable activities. . . . Being in a Discourse is being able to engage in a particular sort of "dance" with words, deeds, values, feelings, other people, objects, tools, technologies, places and times so as to get recognized as a distinctive sort of who doing a distinctive sort of what. Being able to understand a discourse is being able to recognize such "dances."[3]

Although Gee provides a more thorough explanation of Discourse later in his essay, this excerpted summary will do well for our purposes. One may glean from the quote that activists of any kind, if working for societal recognition and respect, may try on the "identity kits" of established institutions. That is, they should abide by particular established Discourses and change things from the inside. Activism, to work with William James's metaphor, will "grow in spots" within established Discourses until they are recognized. Fat activists are doing this and have done it well enough to create a recognizable sub-Discourse of Fat Acceptance. This Fat Discourse has entered the three concepts of Giddens's Structuration theory by utilizing the ready-made "values, beliefs, tools, technologies, and so forth, of Signification, Domination, and Legitimization.

So, what are the values, beliefs, and so forth, of a general Fat Discourse community? Regarding words, fat activists and scholars have coined and shared neologisms that reflect the acts, values, beliefs, and so on that round out Fat Discourse. The following portmanteaus have all become commonplace in Fat Studies and activism: Fatosphere (the online community of Fat Activism, scholarship, and fashion), Fatshion, Fatshionista, Fatkini, fatphobia to name a few. Of course, preexisting concepts like "body politics" are also included.

When discussing the words of Fat Discourse, one must also discuss the words deemed anathema within that Discourse. The terms "Obesity" and "Overweight" are two such words. "Obesity" is shunned because it has developed strong connotations of disease and infirmary. It medicalizes fat in negative ways. "Overweight" is shunned because its meaning is inherently elusive, if not illusory. "*Over*weight" implies a distinctly "normal" weight.[4] If BMI has been debunked as an accurate measure of ideal weight, we have no real gauge of what is our underweight. Thus, the word is jettisoned from the fat lexicon.

Regarding acts, beliefs, attitudes, and social identities, one can look at the behavior of those who have affectively "come out" as fat. These people make a point to wear clothing traditionally deemed only for thin people (think of the fatkini), or nothing at all (think *Adipositivity*). Marie Southard Ospina's video "Redefining Fat," aptly named for our purposes, expresses the outed fatshionista in comprehensive form.[5]

A comprehensive guide to the acts, values, beliefs, attitudes, and social identities inherent in fat Discourse may be Jeanni DePatie and Ragen Chastain's *150 Ways to be a Fat Activist*.[6] This 51-page work is more than just a list of what to do when protesting; it is a sound description of Fat Discourses. DePatie and Chastain categorize activism as working on oneself (cultivating an attitude of self-respect and pride) as well as working for others (an attitude of social justice and critical thinking). Also, activism can be proactive, based on asserting oneself and one's beliefs into the world; or reactive, based on speaking truth to power and battling fat-phobic forces.

This is the "identity kit"[7] of Fat Discourse. One need not do all aspects of it, but familiarity and comfort with all aspects may be imperative to taking on the challenge of Structuration. To be clear, Discourse and Structuration do not share a cause and effect relationship. Discourse has both driven Structuration and has been shaped by it. This is important to realize. In a very real sense, we are raised by societal symbols and their messages, institutions and their ideologies, and policies and their allowances. However, at the same time, all those things were created and are perpetuated or altered by us. Gee's use of dance as a metaphor is an apt one. We dance in and out of—*with*—Discourses, and Discourses dance with us. Recognizing this dynamic is truly an asset for any activist.

NOTES

1. William James, "Pragmatism and Common Sense," *The Writings of William James: A Comprehensive Edition,* ed. By John J. McDermott (Chicago: University of Chicago Press, 1977), 419.

2. Erec Smith, "The Pragmatic Attitude in Fat Activism: Race and Rhetoric in the Acceptance Movement," *The Politics of Size: Perspectives from the Fat Acceptance Movement*, ed. Ragen Chastain (Santa Barbara, CA: Praeger, 2015), 151–162.

3. Marilyn Wann, "Foreward," *The Fat Studies Reader*, ed. Esther Rothblum and Sondra Solovay (New York: New York University Press, 2009), xii.

4. James Gee, *Social Linguistics and Literacies: Ideology in Discourses*, 3rd ed. (New York: Routledge, 2008), 155.

5. "Redefining Fat: Marie Southard Opsina," YouTube.com, 15 March 2015, accessed 2 Nov. 2016, https://www.youtube.com/watch?v=YwF5D0UPEbo.

6. This text was made available to anyone who registered for the 2015 Fat Acceptance Conference.

7. Gee uses the term "identity kit" as a metaphor for one's Discourse.

Bibliography

"About." *Fat People Flipping You Off.* http://fatpeopleflippingyouoff.tumblr.com/about.
"About Let's Move." *Letsmove.gov.* 2013. Accessed 31 Oct. 2016. www.letsmove.gov/about.
Aldebaran and Judy Freespirit. "The Fat Liberation Manifesto." *The Fat Studies Reader*, ed. Esther Rothblum and Sondra Soladay. New York: New York University Press, 2009.
Anderson, Kristen. "Beth Ditto's Clothing Line Is Finally Here!" 12 Feb. 2016. Accessed 30 Oct. 2016. http://www.vogue.com/13398654/beth-ditto-style-clothing-brand-plus-size-fashion/.
Aristotle. *On Rhetoric*. Trans. by George A. Kennedy. New York: Oxford University Press, 2007.
ASDAH. "ASDAH Letter to the House." Association for Size Diversity and Health, Inc. 9 Feb. 2010. Accessed 31 Oct. 2016. https://www.sizediversityandhealth.org/content.asp?id=205&articleID=71.
———. "HAES® Expert DeAun Nelson." Association for Size Diversity and Health. 2016. Accessed 1 Nov. 2016. https://www.sizediversityandhealth.org/haes-expert.asp?id=202.
———. "HAES® Expert Shanti Herzog." Association for Size Diversity and Health. 2016. Accessed 1 Nov. 2016. https://www.sizediversityandhealth.org/haes-expert.asp?id=282.
———. "HAES® Principles." Association for Size Diversity and Health. 2016. Accessed 31 Oct. 2016. https://www.sizediversityandhealth.org/content.asp?id=76.
Bacon, Linda. *Health at Every Size: The Surprising Truth about Your Weight.* Dallas: Benbella Books, 2010. Kindle edition.
Berlin, James. *Rhetoric, Poetics, and Culture: Refiguring College English Studies.* Urbana, IL: NCTE, 1996.
Berthold, Tim and Jill Tregor. "Promoting Healthy Eating and Active Living." *Foundations for Community Health Workers*. 2nd edition, ed. Tim Berthold. San Francisco: Jossey Bass, 2016.
Bias, Stacy. "The 12 Good Fatty Archetypes." Accessed 26 Sept. 2017. http://stacybias.net/2014/06/12-good-fatty-archetypes/.
Bliss, Kelly. Interview, 31 July 2016.
Bordo, Susan. *Unbearable Weight: Feminism, Western Culture, and the Body*. Berkeley, CA: University of California Press, 2003.
Bowers, John W., Donavan J. Ochs, Richard J. Jensen, David P. Schulz, ed. *The Rhetoric of Agitation and Control.* Long Grove, IL: Waveland Press, 2010.
Burgard, Deb. "The HAES® files: Stereotype Management Skills for HBO Viewers." *Health at Every Size Blog.* 8 May 2012. Accessed 28 Oct. 2016. https://healthateverysizeblog.org/2012/05/08/the-haes-files-stereotype-management-skills-for-hbo-viewers/.
Burke, Kenneth. *Language as Symbolic Action.* Berkeley: University of California Press, 1966.

Butler, Judith. *Precarious Life: The Powers of Mourning and Violence*. New York: Verso, 2004.

Campos, Paul, Abigail Saguy, Paul Ernsberger, Eric Oliver, and Glenn Gaesser. "The epidemiology of overweight and obesity: public health crisis or moral panic?" *International Journal of Epidemiology*, 35 (2006).

Campos, Paul. *The Obesity Myth: Why America's Obsession with Weight is Hazardous to Your Health*. New York: Gotham Books, 2004.

Chasmar, Jessica. "Playboy Playmate fired, banned for life from LA Fitness over locker room photo of naked woman." *Washington Post*. 15 July 2016. Accessed 31 Oct. 2016. http://www.washingtontimes.com/news/2016/jul/15/dani-mathers-fired-banned-for-life-from-la-fitness/.

Chastain, Ragen. *Dances with Fat*. Accessed August 3, 2017, https://danceswithfat.wordpress.com/blog/.

———. Email message to author. July 28, 2016.

———. Email to the author. 1 Aug. 2016.

———. "Everybody Galileo Now." *Dances With Fat*. 7 May 2012. Accessed 30 Oct. 2016, https://danceswithfat.wordpress.com/2012/05/07/everybody-galileo-now/.

———. *Fat: The Owner's Manual*. Austin, TX: Sized for Success, 2012.

———. *Ironfat*. Accessed August 3, 2017. https://ironfatblog.wordpress.com/.

———. *The Politics of Size: Perspectives from the Fat Acceptance*. Santa Barbara, CA: Praeger Press, 2015.

———. "A Very Good Place to Start" *Dances with* Fat (blog), June 8, 2015, https://danceswithfat.wordpress.com/2015/06/08/a-very-good-place-to-start/.

Chrisler, Joan and Angela Barney. "Sizism is a Health Hazard." In *The Fat Studies Journal: An Interdisciplinary Journal of Body Weight and Society*. 19 Aug. 2016. Accessed 1 Nov. 2016. doi: 10.1080/21604851.2016.1213066.

Chung, Madelyn. "Playboy Model Dani Mathers Slammed for Publicly Body Shaming Nude Woman at Gym." *Huffington Post*. 15 July 2016. Accessed 31 Oct. 2016. http://www.huffingtonpost.ca/2016/07/15/dani-mathers-body-shaming_n_11015320.html.

Citron, Danielle Keats. *Hate Crimes in Cyberspace*. Cambridge, MA: Harvard University Press, 2014.

Coleman, E Gabriella. "Phreaks, Hackers, and Trolls: The Politics of Transgression and Spectacle." In *The Social Media Reader*. Ed. Mandiberg Michael. New York: New York University Press, 2012. http://www.jstor.org.ezproxy.ycp.edu:8000/stable/j.ctt16gzq5m.12.

Colon, Suzan and Jennifer Traig. *What Would Wonder Woman Do?* San Francisco, CA: Chronicle Books, 2007.

Cooper, Charlotte. "Can a Fat Woman Call Herself Disabled?" *Disability and Society 12*, No. 1, 1997. DOI: 10.1080/09687599727443.

Cuda, Amanda. "Yale Study: Citizens Support Ban of Weight-based Discrimination." *Connecticut Post.* June 27 2010. http://www.ctpost.com/news/article/Yale-study-Citizens-support-ban-of-weight-based-538429.php.

D'Amour, Velvet. "Velvet," *Volup2*. 2015. Accessed 30 Oct. 2016, http://www.volup2.com/velvet/.

"Dances with Facts." Accessed August 3, 2017. https://truthaboutragen.wordpress.com/.

Daufin, E. K. Interview. 20 July 2016. Accessed 2 Oct. 2016. https://www.dropbox.com/home?preview=Ek+Daufin.WAV.

Daniels, Lee. *Wonder Woman: The Golden Age*. San Francisco: Chronicle Books, 2001.

Delacroix, Paul. "Why I Find Supersized Women Beautiful." *BBW_Art.* May 24, 2016, https://bbwart.wordpress.com/paul-delacroix/.

Demello, Margo. *Body Studies: An Introduction.* New York: Routledge Press, 2014.

Doskow, Emily. "Defamation Law Made Easy." *NOLO: Law for All*. 2005. http://www.nolo.com/legal-encyclopedia/defamation-law-made-simple-29718.html.

Erilyn. "Olympians . . . They Come In All Shapes and Sizes." *Fierce, Freethinking Fatties.* Aug 3, 2012, https://fiercefatties.com/2012/08/03/olympians-they-come-in-all-shapes-and-sizes/.

Farrell, Amy. Fat *Shame: Stigma and the Fat Body in American Culture*. New York: New York University Press, 2011.
Fat Activism Conference: Tools for the Revolution. https://fatactivismconference.com/.
Fat Studies Conference, Massey University, 2016, http://www.massey.ac.nz/massey/learning/departments/institute-of-education/events/fat-studies--identity-agency-and-embodiment/fat-studies--identity-agency-and-embodiment_home.cfm.
Fuck Yeah, Fat Haircuts. http://fuckyeahfathaircuts.tumblr.com/.
Gee, James. *Social linguistics and literacies: Ideology in Discourse*. London: Falmer Press, 1990.
Giddens, Anthony. *The Constitution of Society: Outline of the Theory of Structuration*. Berkeley, CA: University of California Press, 1984.
Gladwell, Malcolm. *The Tipping Point: How Little Things Can Make a Big Difference*. New York: Back Bay Books, 2002.
"HAES Matters: Dieting, Disease, and Weight (part 2)" *The Health At Every Size Blog*. 23 Oct. 2012. Accessed 1 Nov. 2016. https://healthateverysizeblog.org/2012/10/23/haes-matters-dieting-disease-and-weight-part-2/.
"Health at Every Size Fact Sheet," Association for Size Diversity and Health (2011).
"How to be fat." *The Sporkful*, Accessed July 28, 2017. http://www.sporkful.com/how-to-be-fat-with-lindy-west/.
Ingeno, Laurent. "Fat-Shaming in Academe." www.insidehighered.com. June 4, 2014.
James, William. "Pragmatism and Common Sense." *The Writings of William James: A Comprehensive Edition*. Ed. By John J. McDermott. Chicago: University of Chicago Press, 1977.
Jones, Substantia. "The Adipositivity Project." Adipositivity.com. Accessed 30 Oct. 2016, http://www.adipositivity.com/
Jones, Substantia. Email message to author, 31 Aug. 2016.
Kirkland, Anna. "What's at Stake in Fatness as a Disability?" *Disability Studies*, 26, No. 1, 2006. http://dsq-sds.org/article/view/648/825.
Lakoff, George. "Understanding Trump." *George Lakoff*. Accessed Aug. 3 2017. https://georgelakoff.com/2016/07/23/understanding-trump-2/.
"Learn the Facts," Let's Move! 2013, accessed, 1 Nov. 2016, http://www.letsmove.gov/learn-facts/epidemic-childhood-obesity.
"Let's Move," Letsmove.gov, 2013, accessed, 31 Oct. 2016 www.letsmove.gov.
Lyons, Pat. "Prescription for Harm: Diet Industry Influence, Public Health Policy, and the 'Obesity Epidemic.'" *The Fat Studies Reader*. Ed. Esther Rothblum and Sondra Solovay. New York: New York University Press, 2009.
Mantilla, Karla. "Gendertrolling: Misogyny Adapts to New Media." *Feminist Studies* 39, no. 2 (2013).http://www.jstor.org.ezproxy.ycp.edu:8000/stable/23719068.
Markham, Edwin. "Outwitted." Poetrynook.com. Accesses 27 July 27, 2018. https://www.poetrynook.com/poem/outwitted.
Mayer, Vivian. "Foreword." *Shadow on a Tightrope: Writings by Women on Fat Oppression*. Ed. By Lisa Schoenfielder and Barb Wieser. San Francisco, CA: Aunt Lute Books, 1983.
Monsma, Bradely John. "'Active Readers . . . Observe Tricksters': Trickster Texts and Cross-Cultural Reading." *Modern Language Studies* 26, no. 4 (1996). doi:10.2307/3195326.
NAAFA. "About Us," National Association for Advancement of Fat Acceptance, Inc. 2016. Accessed 31 Oct. 2016. http://www.naafaonline.com/dev2/about/index.html.
———. "Making the Case for Legislation to End Size Discrimination." National Association of Size Diversity and Health, Inc. 2016. Accessed 31 Oct. 2016. http://www.naafaonline.com/dev2/about/Brochures/NAAFA_Case_for_Legislation_2016.pdf.
———. "NAAFA Newsletter." National Association of Size Diversity and Health, Inc. Sep. 2016. Accessed 31 Oct. 2016. http://www.naafaonline.com/newsletterstuff/oldnewsletter-stuff/September%202016%20NAAFA%20Newsletter.html#LETTER.BLOCK6)ASDAH.
———. "Size-Related Legislation." National Association of Size Diversity and Health, Inc. Accessed 31 Oct. 2016. http://www.naafaonline.com/dev2/about/Policies/Size-Related_Legislation[2015].pdf.
———. "Weight Discrimination Laws," National Association of Size Diversity and Health, Inc., 2016 accessed 31 Oct. 2016. http://www.naafaonline.com/dev2/education/laws.html.

Nichola, Jamar. *BBWW: The Big Beautiful Wonder Woman Blog*. 20 Apr 2012 accessed 30 Oct. 2016. http://fatwonderwoman.blogspot.com/?view=classic.

"Noted Dicks at Tosh.0 Use Stolen Fat-Positive Photo to Make Fun of Fat People," *Jezebel.com* 23 May 2012. Accessed 30 Oct. 2016.http://jezebel.com/5912704/noted-dick-tosh0-uses-stolen-fat-positive-photo-to-make-fun-of-fat-people.

Office of the Surgeon General, "The Surgeon General's Call To Action To Prevent and Decrease Overweight and Obesity," National Center for Biotechnology Information, 2001, accessed 31 Oct. 2016, https://www.ncbi.nlm.nih.gov/books/NBK44206/.

Orbach, Susan. *Fat is a Feminist Issue*. London: Arrow Books, 2006.

Ospina, Marie Southard. "Redefining Fat." *StyleLikeU*. Accessed 26 Sept. 2017. https://www.youtube.com/watch?v=YwF5D0UPEbo.

Paul, Richard. "Critical Thinking in North America." *Critical Thinking: What Every Person Needs to Survive in a Rapidly Changing World*. Tomales, CA: Foundation for Critical Thinking, 2012.

Pausè, Cat. Fuck Yeah, Fat Ph.Ds." *Friends of Marilyn*. June 30, 2015.

Perez, Jessica. "Dani Mathers Should Be Arrested for Policy Violations." Change.org, 2016. Accessed, 31 Oct. 2016. https://www.change.org/p/l-a-county-police-dani-mathers-should-be-arrested-for-privacy-violation.

Phillips, Whitney. *This is Why We Can't Have Nice Things*. Cambridge, MA: MIT Press, 2015.

"Redefining Fat: Marie Southard Opsina," YouTube.com. 15 March 2015. Accessed 2 Nov. 2016. https://www.youtube.com/watch?v=YwF5D0UPEbo.

Rocha, Veronica. "L.A. gym bans Playboy model after she posts body-shaming shower photo on Snapchat." *Los Angeles Times*. 15 July 2016. Accessed 31 Oct. 2016. http://www.latimes.com/local/lanow/la-me-dani-mathers-body-shaming-gym-ban-20160715-snap-story.html.

Rosenberg, Marshall B. *Nonviolent Communication: A Language of Life*. 2nd ed, Encinitas, CA: Puddle Dancer Press, 2003.

Rothblum, Esther. "Why a Journal of Fat Studies?" *The Fat Studies Journal*. Ed. Esther Rothblum. 9 Feb. 2012. Accessed 1 Nov. 2016. http://www.tandfonline.com/loi/ufts20?open=2.

Rothblum, Esther and Sondra Soladay. Ed. by *The Fat Studies Reader*. New York: New York University Press, 2009.

Russell, Constance and Erin Cameron, Ed. *Fat Pedagogy Reader: Challenging Weight-based Oppression Through Critical Education*. New York: Peter Lang Publishing, 2016.

Schopenhauer, Arthur. *The Art of Controversy*. Trans. T. Bailey Saunders. E-book.

Sixel, L. M. "Fired Obese Worker with get $55,000." *The Houston Chronicle*. July 24, 2012. http://www.chron.com/business/article/Fired-obese-worker-will-get-55-000-3732044.php.

Smith, Erec. "By Tort of Defamation: Anti-Fat Campaigns as Civil Wrongs toward People of Size." *Issues: Understanding Controversy and Society*. ABC-CLIO, 2014.

———. "Making Room for Fat Studies in Writing Center Theory and Practice" *Praxis: A Writing Center Journal*. Winter 2013. http://www.praxisuwc.com/smith-101.

———. "The Pragmatic Attitude in Fat Acceptance: Race and Rhetoric in the Fat Acceptance Movement." Santa Barbara, CA: Praeger Press, 2015.

Smucker, Jonathan Matthew. *Hegemony How-To: A Roadmap for Radical*. Chica, CA: AK Press, 2017.

Snider, Stefanie. "'Fat Girls and Size Queens': Alternative Publications and the Visualizing of Fat and Queer Eroto-politics in Contemporary American Culture." *The Fat Studies Reader*. Ed. Esther Rothblum and Sondra Soladay. New York: New York University Press, 2009.

Stern, Marlow. "Meet Ashley Graham, the 'Sports Illustrated' Swimsuit Issue's First 'Plus-Size' Cover Girl," *The Daily Beast*, 17 Feb. 2016. accessed 28 Oct. 2016. http://www.thedailybeast.com/articles/2016/02/17/meet-ashley-graham-the-sports-illustrated-swimsuit-issue-s-first-plus-size-cover-girl.html.

Teagle Consortium. "Liberal Education and Preparation for Life and Work: A Teagle Foundation White Paper." *Teagle Foundation*. 5 Sept. 2008. Accessed 1 Nov. 2016.

Thomas, Pattie. *Taking Up Space: How Eating Well and Exercising Regularly Changed My Life*. Nashville, TN: Pearlsong Press, 2005. Kindle edition.

Tylka, Tracy L. et al. "The Weight-Inclusive versus Weight-Normative Approach to Health: Evaluating the Evidence for Prioritizing Well-Being over Weight Loss." *Journal of Obesity*. 2014. Accessed 1 Nov. 2016. http://dx.doi.org/10.1155/2014/983495.

United States Department of Justice-Civil Rights Division. AMERICANS WITH DISABILITIES ACT OF 1990, AS AMENDED. https://www.ada.gov/pubs/adastatute08.htm#12101.

Vade, Dylan and Sondra Solovay. "No Apology: Shared Struggle in Fat and Transgender Law." *The Fat Studies Reader*. Ed. Esther Rothblum and Sondra Solovay. New York: New York University Press, 2009.

Wahba, Phil. "J.C. Penney Has Tapped This 'Project Runway' Star to Launch Its Plus-Size Brand," *Fortune*. 12 Apr. 2016. Accessed 27 Oct. 2016. http://fortune.com/2016/04/12/jc-penney-project-runway-ashley-nell-tipton/.

Wann, Marilyn. Foreword to *The Fat Studies Reader*. Ed. Esther Rothblum and Sondra Solovay. 1st ed. New York: New York University Press, 2009.

Watkins, Patti Lou, Amy Farrell, and Andrea Doyle Hugmeyer. "Teaching Fat Studies: From Conception to Reception." Oregon State University, April 27 2012, http://oregonstate.edu/instruct/pp/ctla-files/docs/teaching-fat-studies.pdf.

"Weight Discrimination Laws," 2016, http://www.naafaonline.com/dev2/education/laws.html.

Weight of the Nation. HBO, May 2012 access 30 Oct. 2016, http://theweightofthenation.hbo.com/.

West, Lindy. *Shrill: Notes from a Loud Woman*. New York: Hachette Books, 2016.

"What's Underneath," *StyleLikeU*. Accessed 26 Sept. 2017. http://stylelikeu.com/category/the-whats-underneath-project-2/.

Witcombe, Chistopher. "Venus of Willendorf," Art History Resources, 2005, http://arthistoryresources.net/willendorf/.

Witmer, Diane F. "The Construction of Self and Organization: Evoking Organizational Spirituality." *Essays on Communication and Spirituality*. Ed. Amardo Rodriguez. New York: University Press of America, 2001.

Yalom, Irvin D. "Curriculum Vitae." Yalom.com. Accessed 1 Nov. 2016. http://www.yalom.com/pagemaker.php?nav=cv.

———. "Fat Lady," *Loves's Executioner*. New York: Basic Books, 2012.

Index

About the Author

Erec Smith is associate professor of rhetoric at York College of Pennsylvania. His interests in diversity initiatives led him to research on fat activism and the rhetorical tendencies, therein. His other interests include the confluence of rhetoric and Buddhist philosophy and the rhetoric of identity politics.

www.ingramcontent.com/pod-product-compliance
Lightning Source LLC
Chambersburg PA
CBHW071251180926
51613CB00001B/9
9781498531160